Dickie Bar

The
Sterilization
Option

David R. Gober (signature)

The Sterilization Option

A Guide for Christians

David B. Biebel, Editor

Contributors:

Charles K. Casteel
John Jefferson Davis
Joe S. McIlhaney, Jr.
Robert D. Orr
Dean I. Youngberg
Judy Youngberg

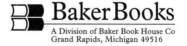

Baker Books

A Division of Baker Book House Co
Grand Rapids, Michigan 49516

Published by Baker Books
a division of Baker Book House Company
P.O. Box 6287, Grand Rapids, MI 49516-6287

Printed in the United States of America

Unless otherwise indicated, Scripture quotations are from the Holy Bible, New International Version®. Copyright 1973, 1978, 1984 by International Bible Society. Used by permission of Zondervan Publishing House. All rights reserved. Other versions used are the King James (KJV).

Except where identified as fictitious, the stories in this book are based on true cases, though the names and some other details have been changed and/or the accounts fictionalized somewhat to enhance readability or to protect the privacy of the individuals involved. Most of the "cases" were written by the editor.

Library of Congress Cataloging-in-Publication Data

The sterilization option : a guide for Christians / David B. Biebel,
    editor : contributors, Charles K. Casteel . . . [et al.].
        p. cm.
    Includes bibliographical references.
    ISBN 0-8010-5267-X (pbk.)
    1. Sterilization (Birth control)—Religious aspects—Christianity.
I. Biebel, David B.
HQ767.7.S83 1995
241'.66—dc20   95-21486

Contents

The opinions expressed in this book are those of the
authors and may not represent the position of any organization with which the authors are,
or have been, associated.

For the name(s) of Christian physicians
(and/or dentists) in your area, contact
the Christian Medical & Dental Society
(615) 844-1000.

Contributors

David B. Biebel, D. Min., has authored five books and collaborated on three others. He is ordained with the Evangelical Free Church of America, and currently serves as Director of Communications for the Christian Medical & Dental Society.

Charles K. Casteel, M.D., has practiced urology since 1964. He lives in Shawnee Mission, Kansas. Dr. Casteel has served as a Trustee of the Christian Medical & Dental Society.

John Jefferson Davis, Ph.D., is Professor of Systematic Theology and Christian Ethics at Gordon-Conwell Theological Seminary in South Hamilton, Massachusetts. He is the author of several books, including *Evangelical Ethics.*

Joe S. McIlhaney, Jr., M.D., is an obstetrician/gynecologist who has practiced in Austin, Texas since 1968. He specializes in the treatment of infertility. Dr. McIlhaney is the author of several books, including *1250 Health Care Questions Women Ask*, and *Safe Sex.*

Robert D. Orr, M.D., is Director of Clinical Ethics at Loma Linda University Medical Center, Associate Professor of Family Medicine at Loma Linda University School of Medicine, and Clinical Co-Director, The Center for Christian Bioethics, Loma Linda University. He co-authored *Life and Death Decisions.*

Dean I. Youngberg, M.D., has practiced internal medicine since 1975. He serves as the chief editor and director for the basic CARE Program, a medical division of the Institute in Basic Life Principles. Dr. Youngberg and his wife, Judy, live in Wichita, Kansas.

1

An Issue with Names and Faces

David B. Biebel
Dean I. Youngberg
Judy Youngberg

Jim and Jenny

When twenty-one-year-old Jim showed up in Dr. Simpson's office, the Christian physician expected the upstanding young man to be concerned about some aspect of his forthcoming marriage. But the doctor never expected to hear him say, "Dr. Simpson, I want a vasectomy."

"Why, Jim? You and Jenny are getting married next month."

"That's why I need a vasectomy."

"But then you wouldn't be able to have any children."

"I know. We're not dumb. We don't *want* to have any children. Pastor Louise says the tribulation is about to begin.

Jenny and I just couldn't bring children into that kind of world. It wouldn't be fair to them."

The physician paused thoughtfully. The young man was certainly sincere. His request was obviously informed, and it seemed to be with his future wife's consent.

As a health care provider, the doctor knew he was free to fulfill the patient's wishes, but as a fellow Christian who was Roman Catholic he could not in good conscience do so. Instead, he tried to change Jim's mind.

"Jim," he said, "a lot of people have predicted the end of the world. And their followers have always been disappointed."

"I don't expect you to understand," Jim replied somewhat angrily, "since you're not one of us. I didn't come here for a sermon. I came for a vasectomy."

"I realize that," the doctor said. "I'm only trying to help you avoid something you'll be sorry for later. Why not use another form of birth control for a while? If you still feel this way in ten years, you can get a vasectomy then."

"I want it now. If you're not going to do it, then send me to somebody who will."

"I'm sorry, Jim. But I'm not willing to do even that, because I'm confident it's not in your best interest to pursue this now."

"I'll let the Lord say what's in my best interest," Jim retorted. "And he speaks through Pastor Louise, not you."

The young man turned on his heel and stalked out.

Depending on your perspective, this true story illustrates good medical ethics in the face of bad theology or bad medical practice in the face of reasonable end-times practical theology.

Either way, it shows how complicated the question of elective sterilization can become for people when religious principles are introduced. Roman Catholics, like Doctor Simpson, have a long history of teachings to guide their perspective and their choices in this matter, as you will see in chapter 4. Protestant denominations, by contrast, have been basically silent on the question of elective sterilization; most leave it up to the conscience of the people involved.

Beyond this, most physicians, including Christian physicians, rely on whatever bioethics they may have learned during their training to guide their practice of things such as elective sterilization. What they would do in Jim's case could largely depend on which current ethical principles guide their medical practice. (The later chapter on medical ethics more thoroughly discusses this.)

Although some doctors might have personal qualms about granting Jim's request, in the end many would do so, assuming the young man was willing to pay the bill. After all, the patient had made an informed, autonomous decision. The doctor had no right to pass judgment on his patient's choice of a permanent form of contraception over the temporary methods available.

Elective sterilization is a growing trend among married Americans. According to research conducted by the National Center for Health Statistics, nearly one in four married women between the ages of fifteen and forty-four has chosen sterilization.[1] Recently the percentage of married men choosing vasectomy also has increased substantially.[2]

These same trends are global. According to the World Health Organization in Geneva, female sterilization is the most widespread form of contraception, accounting for 26 percent of all contraception. Male sterilization accounts for 19 percent, followed by oral contraception at 15 percent.[3]

This increasing use of sterilization as a means of contraception constitutes a significant social phenomenon. Based on these statistics it is likely that many Christian couples have either considered sterilization or have had the procedure. They have done so without much moral guidance, however, since there has been little recent discussion of the pertinent historical, medical, biblical, and ethical dimensions of this crucial issue, especially among evangelical Christians.

Recently, some conservative evangelical leaders have been urging believers who have had sterilizations to seek reversals. This pressure may create considerable confusion and consternation for the couples in question, who probably acted originally in good faith and with a clear conscience. Now, believing that what they did was "sinful," they may be driven by guilt (or the need for approval) to seek a reversal procedure that is medically more difficult and quite expensive (for women, total cost estimates range from $5,000 to $10,000, including hospitalization and anesthesia; for men, from $2,000 to $5,000). It has a high rate of failure (40 percent for women; 55-60 percent for men) and is not usually covered by insurance.

While this book is intended primarily as a guide for couples considering permanent sterilization, it will help couples considering reversal, since the same principles that apply to getting sterilized can also be used to decide whether a reversal would be the action most pleasing to God.

Throughout this book you will find stories of couples who have grappled with the issues under discussion. These stories are only examples, for no two couples are alike and no situation is universal. But they show that voluntary sterilization is not a mere theoretical issue of interest primarily to academicians, theologians, or ethicists. Rather, it is a question with names and faces, people involved in a matter of great significance for the couple, their family, the church, society, the world, and even for the history of the human race, since the birth of a single individual can have implications for all of us.

This book is designed to assist couples who are considering permanent sterilization to make a medically informed, theologically sound, ethically defensible, morally acceptable choice, and to help those who have had sterilization and are considering reversal. It will also help members of the clergy, counselors, and physicians to clarify their thinking on an issue that usually is not given enough advance consideration by most parties involved.

Dave and Ann

Ann and Dave first faced the question of sterilization in 1983 after the birth of their fourth child. Minutes after their daughter was born their Christian family physician asked Ann if she wanted to have her fallopian tubes tied. At that point the procedure would be relatively simple to perform, he explained.

Since the couple had lost one of their two sons to disease five years earlier, Ann declined. "We can try again," she told Dave, "if you want to."

Before that moment, Ann and Dave had not discussed the question of sterilization. Although Dave was an ordained minister, no one had ever asked his advice about this matter, nor had he encountered it during his seminary training. Since he did not know what to say but did know he might like to have another child, Dave agreed that they should not go ahead with the tubal ligation at that time.

Four years later, however, after Ann and Dave learned, through the illness of their second son, that genetic illness stalked their family, the mere thought of fathering another child struck fear in the minister's heart. So he asked the same doctor for information about a vasectomy, which the physician provided with no mention of the Christian ethics involved. Evidently, as far as he was concerned, it was up to Dave.

It never occurred to Dave to seek anyone else's advice, except to ask other men who had had the procedure if they had experienced any unpleasant physical side effects. Still, even though he was encouraged by their responses, the minister could not feel at peace about proceeding. He put it off again.

In 1991, after Dave and Ann had moved two thousand miles west, another Christian doctor suggested it was time for Dave to think about a vasectomy. One concern was to get Ann off "the pill." Beyond that, it was evidently obvious that at age forty-two, Dave would not want to become a father again.

More significant than what this doctor said or implied, however, was what he left out; specifically, that any spiritual, ethical, or moral issues ought to be considered before proceeding with sterilization.

What I have described above was the experience of my wife and me. In our case, the decision-making process was not handled very well, either by us or by the medical professionals involved. Possibly they wrongly assumed we were informed about the religious issues. But our story shows that even when all the parties in a sterilization decision are well-educated, sincere Christians, it is still possible to fail to give all the issues the prayerful consideration and discussion they deserve.

Had we gone ahead without such a process, we might have experienced regrets similar to those expressed by Dean and Judy Youngberg, whose story follows.

My hope is that by hearing about our mistakes you will realize there is a better way to approach this question. At the end of this chapter, I'll offer some suggestions about how to proceed.

Dean's Story

As a young man, my all-consuming priority was to be the top medical student, the leading resident, and ultimately the finest doctor in my field. All of my efforts were directed toward this goal. I even claimed a Scripture verse as verification of my pursuit of excellence in education: "And ye shall know the truth, and the truth shall make you free" (John 8:32 KJV). My erroneous interpretation of this passage was that man's knowledge is the truth. I was in bondage to an educational system dominated by secular humanism. I accepted its philosophies and ignored the only source of all truth: God's Word.

During my medical education, one of the "truths" I accepted was the use of sterilization as a standard procedure for family planning. I readily swallowed the myth of overpopulation.

When my wife, Judy, and I were married, we used several methods of birth control to plan our family, our way. Then, after the birth of our second child, Judy had a tubal ligation.

Soon after I completed medical school and settled into the "comfort zone" of Christian life, God allowed two events to disrupt my prideful, selfish attitude. The first crisis was our firstborn child's grand mal seizure without a known cause at twenty months of age. Several months later, after completing my residency, I was assigned to a one-year, unaccompanied military tour to Southeast Asia. In retrospect, I can see how God used these traumatic experiences to show me I was not the master of my own destiny.

Further conviction came when Judy and I attended a conference, where I heard that God's Word had practical relevance to my medical practice and family. If I claimed to be a child of God, then I needed to give him control over every aspect of my life, including questions of birth control and family size.

This led to an extensive search of Scripture, where I found six purposes for marriage: companionship, pleasure, completeness, protection, illustration of the relationship of Christ and the church, and fruitfulness. The last one has direct impact on the question of sterilization.

Throughout the Bible God uses fruitfulness to indicate his blessing and purpose. God's first command to Adam and Eve involved fruitfulness. "Be fruitful, and multiply, and replenish the earth, and subdue it." (Gen. 1:28 KJV). His instruction was affirmed to Noah after the great flood. "And God blessed Noah and his sons, and said unto them, Be fruitful, and multiply, and replenish the earth" (Gen. 9:1 KJV). The Hebrew words in these verses amplify the meaning of God's commandment concerning abundant fruitfulness. "Be fruitful" means to increase. "Multiply" means to increase exceedingly. "Replenish the earth" means to fill up the world to overflowing. The Lord promised Abraham that his descendants would multiply "as the stars of the heaven, and as the sand which is upon the sea shore" (Gen. 22:17 KJV).

God's design is that his kingdom be advanced through the fruitfulness of his people. This is a physical principle, not only a spiritual one. For example, in Old Testament times, as the nation of Israel grew and multiplied in Egypt, Pharaoh grew alarmed. "And he said unto his people, Behold, the people of the children of Israel are more and mightier than we: Come on, let us deal wisely with them; lest they multiply" (Exod. 1:9,10 KJV).

Pharaoh's strategy to diminish the Israelites' increasing numbers was to exterminate their male newborns. The Hebrew midwives refused to cooperate with the king's plan, however, and God rewarded their courage by blessing them with families of their own.

Today, as then, families that stand for the truth of God's Word pose a great threat to the kingdom of this world, which has mounted a persistent propaganda campaign, intensified during the past three decades. As a result of this campaign, many Christians have embraced the myth of overpopulation and dwindling natural resources and have accepted the idea that they have an obligation to limit their family size. Large families are considered unacceptable and inappropriate. Children are feared, as if they will somehow prevent their parents from achieving "the good life."

When Christian husbands and wives capitulate to this secularistic thinking, they ignore the potential impact a host of righteous sons and daughters could make on our world and thus hinder God from achieving his purposes through their offspring.

We Christians are called to examine our hearts daily to determine the controlling influence of our lives. Are we being swayed by our own desires and the secular philosophies of our day, or are we submitting to God's authority and purpose for our lives? The latter is the only way to please God, as the apostle Paul explained: "For they that are after the flesh do mind the things of the flesh; but they that are after the Spirit the things of the Spirit. For to be carnally minded is death; but to be spiritually minded is life and peace. Because the carnal mind is enmity against God: for it is not subject to the law of God, neither indeed can be. So then they that are in the flesh cannot please God" (Rom. 8:5–8 KJV).

One of the attitudes most pleasing to God must surely be to love children the way he loves them. This positive regard for children is a consistent theme in both Old and New Testaments. For example, the psalmist wrote: "Lo, children are a heritage of the LORD: and the fruit of the womb is his reward. . . . Happy is the man that hath his quiver full of them" (Ps. 127:3,5 KJV).

In the New Testament we see Jesus welcoming and blessing children and chastising his disciples for trying to prevent the children from coming to him. "But Jesus said, Suffer little children, and forbid them not, to come unto me: for of such is the kingdom of heaven" (Matt. 19:14 KJV).

As a result of our study of Scripture relating to fruitfulness, Judy and I came to a crossroads. The Lord pierced our hearts with these soul-searching questions: If I am a sovereign God, is every area of your life and marriage under my control? Do you understand all of my purposes for your marriage, including fruitfulness and loving children?

After considering these questions and experiencing the conviction of the Holy Spirit, we were faced with a crucial decision concerning whether or not we should seek to reverse the tubal ligation Judy had undergone more than a decade earlier.

Judy's Story

When Dean and I were married, we agreed we would have only two children. After all, that was the current ideal family size—in the world's eyes, at least. Our first daughter was born by cesarean section, and when our second child was expected, Dean and I decided to have my tubes tied during the surgery for her birth. Dean asked if I would want to try for a boy should we have another girl, but I said no.

We decided everything our way for our convenience. We did not pray about the decision, ask counsel, or really even consider our actions. We just did it.

Before we decided to try to have children, I had used an intra-uterine device (IUD) to prevent pregnancy. While attending the same conference Dean mentioned, I learned that an IUD prevents pregnancy by not allowing fertilized eggs to implant in the uterus (in other words, an abortion of a developing baby).

I was devastated. I had wanted to control when we had children, and even how many we had, but I certainly had not wanted to kill those the Lord was trying to give us. My heart was greatly broken over what I had selfishly done, even if it was in ignorance. Dean and I both asked God's forgiveness, but I figured that there wasn't anything I could do to reverse things now that I'd been sterilized more than ten years.

A year later we attended another conference. We heard a testimony concerning tubal ligation reversal. I thought that was great for others, but did not seriously consider the issue as it related to me—at least not right away. But occasionally I would wonder how many babies the IUD had aborted, just because I wanted to be in charge of my pregnancies. God continued to work in my heart.

Dean was hesitant to consider a reversal. He did not want us to do this because of pressure from anyone. So I prayed personally, telling God that I was willing to make things right and that I would wait on him to work through Dean.

As the months passed, my heart continued to grieve for the children I had cut off. I prayed for God to do a miracle and allow me to conceive even though my tubes were tied. Deep in my heart, though, I knew it would not happen in my case. Each time my period began, I cried and experienced extreme grief. Finally, I could bear the anguish no longer. I asked Dean for direction, wanting specific guidance either to have a reversal or to leave my body the way it was.

Dean suggested that we search for God's will as a family. He asked our older daughter to find Scripture texts concerning children, birth, and the womb. Our family studied the passages together and found that it is God who opens and closes the womb and that children are a reward from him. Nothing said that a sterilization was pleasing to God. Everything said that God wanted us to have children and populate the earth.

We began a project designed to help discern God's will by a list of questions based on the principles of God's Word. These questions were: What is God's design? What is my responsibility? Whose authority am I under? What suffering will be involved? How is God's ownership acknowledged? What freedom will result? How will true success be seen? The clarity was exciting as we worked our way through and received confirmation for me to have a reversal.

In my personal quiet time I had been reading 2 Kings, observing that very few rulers did what was right in the eyes of the Lord; but many did what was right in their own eyes. A third group sought the Lord but neglected to remove the high places. I realized that I had been taking part in the same iniquity: trying to live righteously, while retaining "the high place" of rejecting more children. It was time to tear down my "high place."

This left us with two matters to be resolved: We had not asked our parents' counsel, nor did we know all the facts about a reversal. When we discussed the matter with our parents, they promised their support, even though they did not understand why we needed to do this.

My gynecologist told us that reversals were his specialty; in fact, his own wife had had one. This doctor was fifty-three years old, and he and his wife were the parents of a four-year-old. He encouraged us to undergo some fertility testing, which we did, with normal results. The only thing left was an exam and other laboratory tests. Everything proved to be favorable.

The Sunday before the surgery, we had a prayer service with the deacons of our church. What a special blessing we

all experienced! God worked in our hearts and gave us his
peace.

Our whole family was very excited about the upcoming
surgery and what it could mean for us. My mother was
worried, fearing that I would die in surgery, but Dean and
my daughters were a tremendous source of strength
throughout the week. God's Word was a constant encour-
agement. I had already given my body to the Lord to do
with as he pleased; I knew that if he chose to take me to
heaven, I was in his hands. I was willing to be obedient,
no matter what the cost.

As I crawled onto the surgery table the morning of the
surgery, I was reminded of Isaac on the altar. Silently I
prayed, "Lord, this is for you. Here is my body. Do with it
as you will." I was at peace.

The surgery lasted a little over four hours. After being
taken to my room, I heard snatches of conversation and
through the sedation pieced together what had happened.
Because the blood supply to my right tube had been cut off,
it was dead. The left tube, however, was fine, so the doctor
had repaired it, saying he had never seen a tube go back
together so perfectly. I began praising and thanking God. I
felt cleansed and whole and pure! It was wonderful! That
entire afternoon and evening we had a worship service right
there in my room. What joy flooded my soul as I rejoiced in
the mighty working of God!

For Dean and me, the lordship of Jesus Christ required
that we yield every area of our life, including our family
size, to him. Personally, by going through with the surgery
I had been obedient to Romans 12: 1, 2 (KJV): "I beseech
you therefore, brethren, by the mercies of God, that ye present your bodies a living sacrifice, holy, acceptable unto
God, which is your reasonable service. And be not con-
formed to this world: but be ye transformed by the renew-
ing of your mind, that ye may prove what is that good, and
acceptable, and perfect, will of God."

How Do You Define Success?

I know you're wondering: How does the story end? Was it all worthwhile? Did the Youngbergs ever produce another child?

That's the way people usually evaluate the "success" of reversals.

But in this case Judy went ahead because she believed that it would be more pleasing to God to give back to him the control of her reproductive life than to retain the control she had taken from him years before. Therefore, her real goal was not to bear as many children as possible but to make it possible for God to give her other children if he saw fit. So far, he hasn't. But that doesn't mean he won't.

The real source of Judy's joy, therefore, is knowing that she has obediently surrendered to God's will. This, ultimately, is the only way to measure success.

Whether or not you agree with her conclusions, it should be obvious that the question of sterilization (or reversal of sterilization) is far more complex than most people realize. This is because it intersects many sensitive areas including personal choice, sexuality, personal values and attitudes, morality, and issues such as guilt, grace, forgiveness, and knowing the will of God—not to mention doing it.

One common approach to all this complexity is to say that since the Bible does not specifically address elective surgical sterilization, no one should force a particular meaning on the silence of God. Many evangelicals, possibly a majority, believe that elective sterilization, like many other modern issues, is a matter of conscience best left between an individual (or couple) and God—an arena into which no other person (or institution) should intrude.

The problem for couples trying to make a God-honoring choice about sterilization (or reversal) is that this lack of guidance may leave them free to choose sterilization while also leaving them vulnerable later, especially if their choice is challenged by someone who seems to have superior spiritual insight on the matter.

The most responsible approach, therefore, is not to blindly adopt anyone's position—even the position that there is no correct position—but to search the Scripture yourself with an open mind and heart. Ask the Holy Spirit to enlighten you and help you to apply what you find to your own situation in such a way that whatever choice you make, you will have God's peace.

Remember the general principles that apply when sincere believers differ. Allow me to expand a bit what the apostle Paul told a group of believers who were debating the questions of whether or not a Christian could, with a clear conscience, eat meat that had been sacrificed to idols.

"It all comes down," Paul says, "to the question of faith. One person can eat the meat because his faith is strong and he knows idols are nothing. Another abstains because it evokes memories of the pagan rites, and therefore violates his conscience. In neither case should one judge the other, for to his own master (the Lord) he must stand or fall. As far as I'm concerned, no meat is unclean in itself. But if anyone regards something as unclean, then for him it is unclean. In this case, the one who doubts but goes ahead anyway is violating his conscience because he is not acting in faith; and everything that does not come from faith is sin" (see Romans 14).

The purpose of this book is to help you act in faith in relation to elective sterilization or reversal. In other words, how you proceed will be based on humble and obedient surrender to God's will as you understand it. In this context, an unfaithful decision would be to go ahead, even though you are not fully convinced. Or, it might mean to pursue a reversal because of guilt heaped on you by someone else.

Further, your behavior might reflect an attitude of superiority because you think you understand this issue better than someone else, or perhaps indifference, as if your perspective and how you act on it has no personal or spiritual significance, without actually examining for yourself if this is so.

The rest of this book is designed to help you formulate a medically informed, theologically sound, ethically defensible, morally acceptable position about voluntary sterilization. After that, the only issue left will be whether or not you will faithfully put into practice what you believe, striving to please the only master to whom you must answer.

For Reflection or Discussion

Jim and Jenny

1. Role play the following situation: Jim and Jenny, still unmarried, have postponed sterilization pending a meeting with Pastor Louise, who has invited Dr. Simpson to attend.

2. To see how complicated the question of elective sterilization can become, following the role play have the participants debrief (with the help of their audience). Have them try to separate the issues into categories such as medical, ethical, sexual, spiritual/religious, emotional, moral, legal.

3. What do you think Jim and Jenny should do?

    ___ Use other methods of pregnancy prevention for a while after they are married.
    ___ Find a different church.
    ___ Find a different doctor.
    ___ Whatever they think is best.
    ___ Stop involving others in what is a purely personal matter.
    ___ Ask their parents for advice.
    ___ Ask their grandparents for advice.
    ___ Get a puppy and wait for the tribulation to begin.
    ___ Discuss this with a couple who have been sterilized.
    ___ Other

4. Role play, having Jenny and Jim discuss their plan privately as they sit in their car in the church's parking lot following the meeting.

Dave and Ann

1. If you believe that Dave and Ann's range of acceptable options differs from that of Jim and Jenny, identify the reasons:

   ___ They are too old to raise any more children.
   ___ More children might cause undue hardship.
   ___ They already have had four children, a "full quiver" by anybody's standards.
   ___ Based on their genetic history, they have a moral obligation not to have more children.
   ___ They have a moral obligation before God to produce as many offspring as possible.
   ___ They are free before God to do whatever they believe is best.
   ___ Dave should follow the second doctor's advice and stop leaving the entire burden on Ann.
   ___ Other

2. Why, do you think, the question of voluntary sterilization is not frequently or openly discussed in the church or Christian literature?

   ___ It's a purely personal issue.
   ___ People don't want advice about it.
   ___ People are embarrassed to ask for advice about it.
   ___ It's irrelevant to faith and/or spirituality.
   ___ The Bible has nothing to say about it.
   ___ It's not really an issue except for people who write books like this.
   ___ Other

Dean and Judy

1. The Youngbergs concluded that having a reversal would be more pleasing to God than leaving things the way they were. Suppose you were their close friend, and either of them had sought your advice about this conclusion. What would you have said?

2. Having read this chapter, try to write a rough draft of your position on voluntary sterilization. You do not have to resolve every aspect of this question for now.

3. What main point have you seen in this chapter?

2

Medically Informed

Female Sterilization

Joe S. McIlhaney, Jr.

Mary

Mary was only twenty-four when she asked her doctor to sterilize her. Since she was already the mother of two children, and her husband seemed to be in hearty agreement, I did a double-puncture laparoscopic sterilization (see the description of methods below). The procedure required two small incisions, general anesthesia, and about twenty minutes to perform. There were no medical complications. Unresolved issues between Mary and her husband led to their divorce two years later.

Mary's second husband was willing to help raise the children, who were still living with her, but he wanted to father one or two of his own. After extensive evaluation, we determined that Mary's fallopian tubes could not be repaired.

The couple's only alternative was in vitro fertilization, which was beyond their means.

Looking back, Mary acknowledged that she really had been too young and immature when she made the earlier decision. She had consented to have the procedure under pressure from her first husband, who had wanted no more than two children.

The Most Common Reasons for Female Sterilization

If a woman has a medical problem, such as heart disease or severe diabetes, that makes it dangerous for her to become pregnant, her doctor may recommend sterilization. Wife, husband, and doctor reach a joint decision to avoid pregnancy under these circumstances. Fortunately, these life-threatening conditions are unusual.

A genetic problem that dramatically increases the possibility of having an abnormal child is another medical reason to consider sterilization. Before a couple has a sterilization for this reason, I advise them to seek expert genetic counseling.

Occasionally a woman will want sterilization because she dislikes other methods of contraception. Because of its relative permanence, however, I strongly feel this is not an adequate reason for sterilization. It should be done because a woman never wants another child. Compared with the devastation she may face when she realizes after sterilization that she wants another child, a little inconvenience with a birth control method is a minor issue.

Some women choose sterilization so that they can pursue a career, then change their minds later. I have seen this happen many times. If a woman has no children but feels she wants a career instead, I urge her not to have a sterilization procedure until she is in her forties.

Statistics show that people under age thirty who have a sterilization are more likely to want that sterilization reversed later. Persons in this age group considering sterilization should be particularly cautious before they make the final decision to have the procedure performed. If they have any doubts about their decision, they should not have it done.

Many women let fear of pregnancy frighten them into having a sterilization. Again, the basic reason for sterilization should be the decision never to have more children, not fear of becoming pregnant. Reliable pregnancy prevention methods are available which allow normal fertility when discontinued.

Some women have a sterilization done during a time of upheaval in their lives. Commonly this is during divorce proceedings or within a year or two after divorce. Because such situations are very stressful and emotional, not good times to make any major decisions, it is better to wait until later when things have settled down.

Sterilization Procedures

From my perspective I believe it is better for the woman than the man to have the sterilization. It is she whose body bears the risks inherent in pregnancy. If she is sterilized, she no longer has to worry about the risk, even if she loses her husband by divorce or death and later remarries. However, if her former husband rather than she has the sterilization, and she then enters into a new marriage, she must consider again what she wants to do about her fertility.

Tubal Ligation

Tubal sterilization, or tubal ligation, is now the most common method of sterilization for women in the United States. The procedure blocks the fallopian tubes so that an egg from the ovaries cannot pass through them to be potentially fertilized. If the tubes are closed, a woman normally cannot get pregnant.

There are several different ways to have a tubal ligation, but all require some type of surgery.

An interval sterilization is one performed at some time other than immediately following a delivery. It is usually accomplished through small abdominal incisions, using either laparoscopic or minilaparotomy techniques.

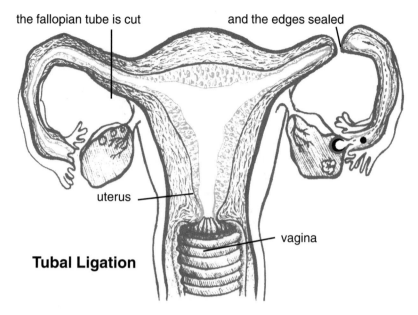

the fallopian tube is cut   and the edges sealed

uterus

vagina

Tubal Ligation

Laparoscopy sterilization is the most commonly used technique for sterilizing women today. It is performed with the help of a special viewing instrument called a laparoscope that is inserted into the abdomen. Since it is not major surgery, the patient can usually go home from the hospital the same day the laparoscopy is performed. The procedure can occasionally be done with a local anesthetic, but general anesthesia is normally used. Laparoscopy is sometimes called "Band-Aid" surgery, because the incisions can be covered by Band-Aids.

To do this surgery, the doctor dilates the cervix, inserts an instrument into the uterus, and lifts it. A small needle is inserted into the lower edge of the umbilicus (navel), through which two or three quarts of carbon dioxide gas are introduced into the abdomen. This lifts the wall of the abdomen off the intestines, so the operating instruments can be safely inserted into the abdominal cavity.

Most doctors use a technique that requires two incisions. One (about one-third inch long) is made just above the pubic bone,

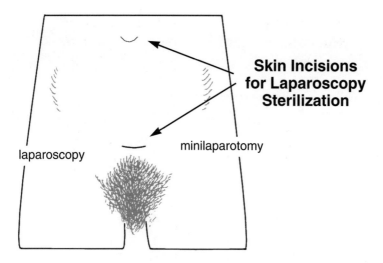

**Skin Incisions
for Laparoscopy
Sterilization**

laparoscopy   minilaparotomy

and the other (about a half-inch long) is made in the lower edge
of the navel. A small amount of pubic hair may need to be
shaved for the lower incision. The laparoscope is inserted
through the higher incision, and through it the doctor observes
the pelvic structures. The instruments are inserted through the
lower incision.

After the fallopian tubes have been blocked by either cautery,
clip, or band (described below), the instruments are removed, the
gas is allowed to escape, and the incisions are closed.

In cautery and division the tubes are cauterized to keep them
from bleeding when they are cut. Then each tube is cut through
where the burn was made, usually about a third of the way from
the uterus to the end of the tube.

Hulka clips are small clips with copper springs. They are placed
over the middle part of the tube and closed. Pressure keeps the
blood flow from going through the part of the tube inside the
clip. That part of the tube dies, effectively blocking the tube.

A Falope ring is a rubber band-shaped piece of silicone that is
put around a "knuckled-up" portion of the tube. Such a ring is
so tight that it cuts off the blood supply, which causes the part of
the tube it encircles to die and thus divides the tube.

Hulka spring clip

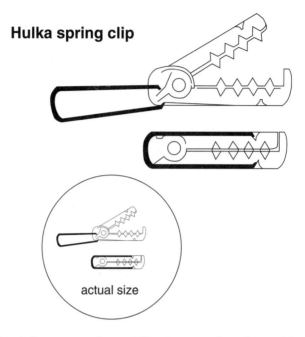

actual size

A minilaparotomy is a sterilization procedure done without the laparoscope. Only one incision is made, slightly larger than for a laparoscopy, just above the pubic bone. Using an instrument inserted into the uterus, the doctor pushes the uterus up against the wall of the abdomen just under the incision. With small instruments the doctor reaches into the incision, pulls the fallopian tubes up through the hole, and then ties and cuts them. This procedure usually is done under general anesthesia, though it is possible to do it with a local.

Years ago doctors did sterilizations through the vagina. This required general anesthesia and an incision in the upper vagina, right behind the cervix. The doctor would pull the fallopian tubes down far enough to tie and cut them. The procedure allowed a woman to have a sterilization done without a larger incision in the abdomen.

However, this was not a reliable method of sterilization. The doctor was often unable to find both fallopian tubes after making the colpotomy incision and had to make a large abdominal

Minilaparotomy

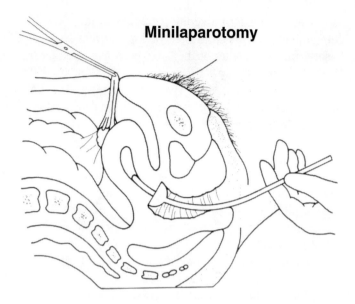

incision to complete the procedure. There was a greater chance of infection with vaginal surgery, because the vagina cannot be made as clean for surgery as can the skin of the abdomen.

These days the large abdominal incision method is outdated and unnecessary. If a surgeon says the procedure requires a larger than one-inch abdominal incision, find a doctor who will do either a minilaparotomy or a laparoscopy sterilization. A vaginal tubal ligation should be considered only if it is impossible for the wife to have a laparoscopy.

Postpartum Sterilization

A postpartum sterilization is one that is done immediately after delivery of a baby, or during the next day or two. If a couple knows for sure this baby is the last child they want to have, it is convenient and sensible to have the sterilization done immediately after the delivery. The sterilization can be done following either a normal vaginal delivery or a cesarean section.

The only warning I give my patients considering this procedure is that the baby's life is at the highest risk during the first twenty-four hours after birth. A newborn may seem normal but die within the first day because of some abnormality which was impossible to detect at birth. This happens rarely, but if a couple would want another child if their newborn were to die, they should delay sterilization at least a day or two. It would be even wiser to wait about six months.

Immediately after a vaginal delivery the uterus is still quite large. The top of it is usually at the level of the navel, making the fallopian tubes, which are attached to the top of the uterus, easily accessible through a small incision in the lower edge of the navel. The doctor merely makes a single incision, reaches in first to one side and then the other, picking up each fallopian tube separately and pulling it through the incision so it can be tied and cut. The small incision is then closed with sutures.

Sterilization immediately after a cesarean section is the easiest of all sterilizations to do. After sewing up the uterus, the doctor merely reaches over, lifts each tube with a clamp, ties it with a suture, and cuts away the part of the tube that has been tied off.

Emotional Reactions

Women occasionally have emotional difficulty dealing with a sterilization, but this does not seem to have a physical cause. Studies show that from 2 to 4 percent of women regret having had a sterilization. Usually, these are women who had the procedure done when they were young and were childless, or had only one or two children. In spite of this regret, only two women per thousand actually have their tubes put back together later.

Medical Risks

Any surgical procedure carries risks. Before any type of surgery, a patient should understand the potential dangers that can accompany an operation. The potential problems associated with a sterilization procedure include:

> Damage to the intestines, which could necessitate major surgery, even a colostomy.
>
> Bleeding into the abdomen, which could require a large incision so the surgeon could locate the bleeding vessel and suture it. The bleeding could also lead to the need for a blood transfusion, which may result in developing hepatitis or other diseases.
>
> Infection in the abdomen, which could cause a life-threatening abscess that could make a hysterectomy mandatory.
>
> Death from complications of either the anesthetic or the surgery.

These dangers could scare a woman if she did not realize that not being sterilized, and then using a less reliable method of birth control, exposes her to the dangers of pregnancy, which are greater than those of sterilization. About 1.5 out of 100,000 women who have a sterilization procedure will die as a result of it. By comparison, approximately 7.8 per 100,000 women die of complications related to pregnancy.

What Happens to Eggs and Sperm After Sterilization

Following sterilization both the egg and any sperm that enter the cervix die inside a woman's body. The egg usually dies within twenty-four hours after ovulation, and most sperm will be dead within two or three days after entering the woman's body. After the cells die, a very little protein residue is absorbed into the body. Millions of cells in a person's body die and are absorbed and replaced every day. The absorption of dead egg and sperm cells is no different and does not damage a woman's body.

Sterilization does not seem to negatively affect a wife's interest in or practice of sex with her husband.

Some studies suggest possible increased risk of menstrual disturbance in women who have had a sterilization, but that is not likely to occur until at least two years after the sterilization. Any irregularity of the menstrual periods prior to two years is not a result of the sterilization procedure.

Some experts claim that women who have been sterilized have increased risk for a later hysterectomy. Several factors may indicate the need for a hysterectomy. Perhaps women who have had a sterilization have had more children than women who have not had a sterilization, and the damage to the reproductive organs of a woman who has had several babies can cause her to need a hysterectomy for repair of that damage. Also, women who have had sterilization and later have a reproductive organ problem may be more likely to have a hysterectomy that, although not mandatory, can be beneficial. Although there is no indication that tubal sterilization damages a woman's uterus, the increased bleeding some women have after a sterilization might cause the need for a future hysterectomy in a few women.

The Centers for Disease Control have not yet completed a study begun in 1978 which will evaluate the effects of sterilization on women's bodies. The study will probably help resolve the question of whether or not sterilization is damaging to a woman's body.

Reversal of Sterilization

Even though couples are warned before they have a sterilization to be sure they never want another child, many change their minds about having another child after a few years.

Several situations may be associated with a woman's desire to be pregnant again: new marriage partner, death of an infant or child, desire for more children, change in sexual responsiveness, or emotional feelings after sterilization.

For example, Cynthia had her tubes tied after Gretchen, her second child was born. Cynthia and John, her husband, were sure they would not want to have any more children. But they didn't investigate all the possibilities. Tragically, Gretchen crawled under the couch one day, found a plastic bag, put it on, and suffocated. Cynthia returned to me, hoping we could repair her tubes. Fortunately for her and John, the operation was a success and they are now the parents of three children.

This brings up a final but very important factor to be considered. Repair of the fallopian tubes requires a major operation and an expense of several thousand dollars. Then, after all that, there is no guarantee that a pregnancy will result. Only 50 to 75 percent of women become pregnant after their tubes are repaired. Thus 25 to 50 percent will still not become pregnant after such surgery.

If a woman's sterilization results in destruction of most of her fallopian tubes or the destruction of the fimbriated (outer) ends of the tubes, it will be difficult, or even impossible, for a gynecologic microsurgery to allow the woman a very good chance of pregnancy.

The most successful fallopian tube repairs are those in which the fimbriated ends of the tubes and most of both tubes are still intact. If at least two and a half to three inches of tube are left after the repair has been completed, the chances of pregnancy are increased.

Male Sterilization

Charles K. Casteel

Seventeen-year-old Julian surprised me. "I want a vasectomy," he said.

"Why?" I asked. "You're not married. If you ever got married, you wouldn't be able to have any children."

"I know," he shrugged his shoulders. "But my father says I have to have this done."

"Why?"

"Because I already got three girls pregnant," Julian replied. "He thinks I'm gonna keep doing that."

"Are you?"

"Maybe," the boy said. "It all depends on the girl."

"Don't you think the responsibility is yours, too?"

"Not really. I'm addicted to sex. But she doesn't have to say yes. Now, are we going to do this or not?"

"I can't do it, in good conscience. Besides, I don't think it's a good idea. You'll be sorry later. You may be old enough to get people pregnant, but you're not mature enough to make this decision. However, I would like to talk to your father."

The first human vasectomy was performed by Reginald Harrison in 1893. During the first century of this procedure's history, the understanding of its effects and the reasons for doing it have frequently been confused and misguided. Early on there were theories, supported mostly by anecdotal reports, of its effectiveness in preventing or curing benign prostatic hypertrophy, a commonly occurring enlargement of the prostate gland. The procedure was thought to sexually rejuvenate elderly men. By the year 1936, "the number of 'scientific' publications describing its effects had exceeded 1,000, and many thousands of vasectomies had been performed for these purposes."[1]

On the darker side, this simple sterilization procedure was misapplied. In 1899, for example, A. J. Ochsner recommended the practice of sterilizing habitual criminals to prevent their passing on "certain inherited anatomic defects which characterize these men."[2] Ochsner broadened his recommendation when he said that "the same treatment could be reasonably suggested for chronic inebriates, imbeciles, perverts and paupers."[3]

From 1934 to 1945 up to one million vasectomies were performed in Nazi Germany, mainly for what they claimed would be race improvement.

In the early 1900s through the 1960s, a legitimate use of vasectomy during prostate surgery was done to prevent epididymitis. This is no longer routine because of newer approaches to prostate surgery and the availability of effective antibiotics.

Today the major use of vasectomy is for voluntary sterilization—no promises or evidence of sexual rejuvenation, no forced submission to genetic promises or threats, no political or social coercion. No one can force anyone to be sterilized today, which is why I refused to accommodate Julian's father, even though I was sympathetic with his concern.

In the United States, approximately 500,000 men undergo vasectomy each year. Nearly 7 percent of all married couples choose vasectomy as their form of birth control. Obviously, in a relatively short time this simple procedure has become quite popular for men who wish permanently to eliminate their reproductive ability.

Patient Selection

I believe that ideally vasectomy should be considered only within marriage. The decision should be mutual. If husband or wife has serious reservations regarding permanent sterilization it is best postponed until all the issues have been resolved. A husband should not have a vasectomy if his wife is reluctant, nor should he be pressed into a procedure which he either does not want or fears. This procedure should not be undertaken if there is any thought on the part of the couple that they might want more children in the future. Although reversal of vasectomy is possible, it carries such a high rate of failure (55-60 percent) that vasectomy should never be considered a temporary option.

There are no hard and fast rules as to the age of the couple requesting vasectomy nor the number of children they already have, or if they have children. Sterilization calls for responsible decision making and obviously can be abused by those who fail to be responsible.

It is the responsibility of the physician to help facilitate well-informed, mutually agreed-upon decisions but not to dictate or take sides if there is lack of agreement.

Surgical Technique

The vas deferens is a muscular tube approximately thirty-five centimeters long and three millimeters in diameter. It extends from the tail of the epididymis upward through the scrotum to

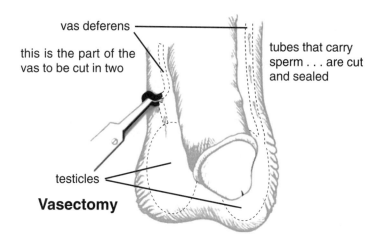

vas deferens

this is the part of the vas to be cut in two

tubes that carry sperm . . . are cut and sealed

testicles

Vasectomy

the region of the prostate, where it joins the duct of the seminal vesicle to form the ejaculatory duct. It is composed of three layers of smooth muscle capable of powerful contractions, which help propel sperm along its length.

Although there are several variations on the technique, the basic vasectomy procedure is usually carried out in the doctor's office or an outpatient facility using local anesthesia. In most cases this is accomplished with minimal discomfort.

The vas is isolated immediately under the skin of the scrotum, a small incision or puncture wound is made, and the small tube is lifted out. A segment of approximately one centimeter is excised. The two ends of the vas are then closed off with either surgical clips, sutures, cautery, or a combination of these. The ends are then allowed to slip back into the scrotum and the skin edges are sutured if necessary.

The local anesthetic will usually last for an hour or so to allow the patient to return home. A mild analgesic is administered as needed for pain, and an ice pack is used intermittently the first twenty-four hours. Patients should avoid heavy exertion for forty-eight hours.

After a vasectomy, some sperm will remain in the connected portion of the vas. It is therefore necessary to continue to use effective contraceptives until fifteen or twenty ejaculations have occurred and for about six weeks, the time it takes to complete healing and scarring over of the ends of the vas. At the end of that time, semen specimens must be checked until at least two consecutive specimens are free of sperm. This is to confirm the absence of any sperm in the ducts and to be sure there has been no spontaneous recanalization or regrowth of the vas where it was severed.

Immediately following a vasectomy there may be a mild ache, mild bruising of the scrotal skin, and mild swelling. These are expected and should not be considered unusual. The patient may resume sexual activity as soon as he feels comfortable, with the stipulation that contraceptives are used until two negative semen specimens are completed.

Results of Vasectomy

The effect of vasectomy is to prevent sperm from reaching the area of the prostate and seminal vesicals. Most of the fluid which is expressed as ejaculate comes from these structures. There are no changes in the sexual responses or sexual desire.

Medical Risks

The statistical incidence of medical complications of vasectomy is about 1 to 2 percent. These are usually minor and include skin infections, bleeding into the scrotum, and leakage of sperm into the scrotum or congestion of the epididymis by sperm which cannot be ejaculated. It is unusual for these problems to be of more than minor inconvenience. They should respond to treatment in a short time.

Through the years, concerns have been raised about whether there might be unexpected or unknown complications from vasectomy. In the 1970s concern about autoimmune phenomena was dispelled by scientific study. In the early 1980s there was concern about potential heart risks in vasectomized men. Again, several broad public health studies resolved those issues. More recently, in February 1993, published statistical surveys suggested a possible link between vasectomy and prostate cancer. Although some time will need to elapse before definitive answers can be stated, numerous current studies indicate that there is no strong cause and effect relationship between vasectomy and prostate cancer.

Psychological Risks

As far as I can tell, most of my patients have not experienced adverse psychological reactions following their surgery. Unless I missed something in follow-up visits, nearly all of them were satisfied with both their decision and the results of the procedures. If anything, they usually expressed a clear sense of relief that they could no longer father a child, especially "by mistake."

But it is possible that my patients have been reluctant to share with me the kind of emotional turmoil following sterilization that one Christian we'll call Tony experienced:

Tony and Susan's fourth child was stillborn, at nineteen weeks gestation. "The baby looked like a tiny white crane that had washed up on shore," Tony said. "We sent a snip from its patella tendon to the Mayo Clinic, to determine if the miscarriage was due to a genetic problem."

Although they never got an answer to the genetic question, less than six months later the couple decided they would not want to have any more children. Tony decided to get a vasectomy because it was, in his words, "more fair, and less risky."

The procedure proved more painful and difficult than Tony had expected. "The doctor lost one of the vas ends," Tony recalled, "and had to go looking for it. Beyond that trauma, after the surgery I had quite a lot of bleeding," he added.

But more surprising to Tony than the doctor's ineptitude was his own reaction. "It upset me in some ways that I had this done," he said. "Not so much that I could no longer cause pregnancy, since that was why I'd had it done," he added. "Occasionally I had regrets that we would have no more children. More than that, there was the sense that I was no longer a young man. It seemed I had irreversibly passed a phase in life and I was no longer in my prime."

During this unsettled period, Tony also struggled with sexual thoughts and masturbation, even some attraction to pornography, very unlike his normal patterns of thinking and acting. In retrospect, Tony believes this reaction was due to his anxiety about whether or not his sexual functioning had been altered by the surgery.

"In talking with other men about this," he said, "many have expressed the same kinds of concerns and conflicts about sexual function. Fortunately," he added, "I did not act this out with another woman. But I can see how some men might even end up having an affair in order to prove something to themselves."

Obviously, temporary psychological reactions are possible when a person's sexual functioning has been altered. And it would be helpful for men considering sterilization to anticipate facing the kinds of issues Tony mentions, so they don't end up "having an affair in order to prove something to themselves."

Conclusion

Despite vasectomy's potential side effects, once a couple has decided that it is time for one of them to be sterilized, I believe that vasectomy has numerous advantages over tubal ligation, including simplicity, lower cost, avoidance of abdominal procedures, use of local anesthesia, and, perhaps most important, an easy way to assess its effectiveness. In that small number of men in whom recanalization may occur (estimated at 1 per 1000), this can be readily recognized. For women, the risk of tubal recanalization is approximately the same, but this is discovered only by subsequent pregnancy, an obviously more serious consequence.

Even if it weren't for its other advantages, I believe that this last one is reason enough to conclude that for couples who have made a mature decision to seek sterilization, vasectomy is preferable to female sterilization in most cases.

For Reflection or Discussion

1. In Mary's case, what could have been done differently to help the young woman avoid the situation she eventually faced?

    ___ Mary might have told the doctor about her husband's coercion.

___ The doctor might have suggested that she wait.
(If you choose this one, how long is long enough?)
___ Mary could have told her husband to get sterilized, since it was his idea.
___ Mary and her husband could have gotten some advice from their pastor.
(If you choose this one, what advice do you think they would have received?)

2. Without consulting the following chapters, rate the following reasons for sterilization in terms of degree of acceptability. Use a 1–10 rating system, 10 being unquestionably okay and 0 being highly questionable.

   (Note: If you are studying in a group, do not try to reach consensus on these at this point. Also, keep in mind that some in your group may have already been sterilized for one or more of the reasons given.)

   ___ The woman has a medical condition that might be dangerous to her if she became pregnant.
   ___ There is a family history of genetic disease.
   ___ Other methods of birth control are inconvenient.
   ___ Children might hinder either person's career.
   ___ The couple can't afford more children (or even one child).
   ___ The couple has as many children as they want.
   ___ Some people have suggested the couple has enough children already.
   ___ The world is overpopulated.
   ___ It's not fair to bring children into these "end times."
   ___ An unmarried minor has already produced several illegitimate children.

3. Discuss the case of Cynthia and John, and on the basis of their experience, develop some practical advice about sterilization for young couples.

4. Role play the discussion between Dr. Casteel and Julian's father. Identify the basic issues for Julian, his father, and Dr. Casteel.

5. Decide if Dr. Casteel was justified in refusing to sterilize Julian. If so, list all your reasons under these categories: medical, theological, ethical, moral, other.

6. In this chapter, the obstetrician/gynecologist favors sterilization for women, and the urologist favors sterilization for men. Which do you think has the strongest position, and why?

3

Ethically Defensible

Robert D. Orr

Darcy and Walter

Darcy and Walter are well-educated, career-oriented, and childless. After ten years of marriage, they are considering sterilization so they can both be professionally fulfilled.

They go to see a local Christian family physician, who knows them well and attends the same church they do. The doctor says she might be willing to help them, but only if the couple will resolve one question before they proceed.

"On what basis have you made this decision?" the doctor asks.

Walter looks at Darcy, then back to the doctor. "On the basis that we know what we want," he offers.

"And what we don't want," Darcy adds.

"I can see that," the doctor replies. "And for a lot of my patients, that's all that matters. They think they are the masters of their own destinies."

The doctor pauses, looking her friends in the eye, then adds, "But I know you both well enough to know your view of the world is different from that."

"True enough," Walter replies. "But what does faith have to do with this?"

"Everything," the doctor says, "or nothing. It's up to you to decide."

In twenty-five years as a family doctor, I have participated in scores of sterilizations. But seldom have I had the kind of conversation illustrated by this fictitious case. I refused to sterilize single individuals. But if sterilization was something the patient and spouse were sure they wanted, and they were properly informed of the risks, I felt free to provide the service. Only rarely did anyone ask my advice regarding the ethics of their decision.

Had I been asked, I don't know what I would have said, since very little was taught about this in medical school or in other aspects of my training, where sterilization was presented as an acceptable alternative form of pregnancy prevention. Modern surgical techniques had made sterilization procedures safe and convenient enough, but trustworthy guidance on what should be done was remarkably absent.

Had it addressed the issue, the field of medical ethics could have provided some guidance. Since you may not be familiar with this field, let me briefly review the history of medical ethics and especially how it has developed over the past three decades.

Ethics is the branch of applied philosophy which deals with values as they relate to human conduct. It deals with good and bad, right and wrong, vice and virtue, and attempts to answer the question, "What should be done?"

Medical ethics relates these values to the practice of medicine. Questions of medical ethics have become more common and more difficult in recent years because of advancing technology, a changing doctor-patient relationship, the urgency of cost containment, and perhaps other reasons.

Modern medical ethics began in the 1960s when theologians began to point out to clinicians that in situations without clear answers they should ask, "What should we do?" rather than, "What can we do?" So, modern medical ethics was initiated by individuals concerned about religious values. However, we hear little about religious values in discussions about medical ethics today. Medical ethics has been secularized, and not for nonreligious people only.

A Question of Perspective

Even religious people like Walter and Darcy often make their medical decisions without asking how faith-related components should guide them. As this couple admitted, when they made their initial decision, it was on the basis of what they wanted. In other words, as they viewed it, the main issues were centered on them—their needs, desires, dreams—and they believed that they had the authority to choose what they thought best.

This human-centered (anthropocentric) approach excludes external authority or guidance, except perhaps when it considers legal, social, or moral traditions of whatever society the decision makers are part of.

Their doctor, by contrast, suggested that since they are believers, their view of the world, or worldview, is different. In the Christian worldview, God is central. God has authority. God has control. God gives guidance. The individual has been created in the image of God (*Imago Dei*), but is living in a fallen state and is in need of redemption. Guidance for decision making for the individual Christian comes from God's revealed Word and the ongoing work of the Holy Spirit. The individual receives this guidance through prayer, searching Scripture, and counsel from other believers.

If Walter and Darcy are to answer their doctor's question about the basis of their decision, they must decide to what degree they are willing to allow their Christian worldview to affect their decision regarding sterilization.

To further complicate matters, they also need to know that their worldview is only one component of the process. If it were the only component, secularists and Christians would nearly always disagree. The reason they don't always disagree is because people from differing perspectives may use similar theories of moral reasoning to reach health care decisions.

Theories of Moral Reasoning

There are several theories of moral reasoning, but the dominant theory used in medical ethics in recent decades is that specific decisions can be made by applying well-recognized principles. This theory is called principlism.

Four basic principles of medical ethics are widely accepted by secularists today.[1] The first two—doing good for patients (beneficence) and "first of all, do no harm" (non-maleficence)—have their origins in antiquity and have been accepted and practiced for centuries. They form the basis for the broad goal of medicine to relieve suffering.

The third principle, the right to self-determination (autonomy) is a rather new concept in medicine. Until thirty years ago, it was common and expected for physicians to do what they thought best for patients without necessarily involving them in the decision-making process. Declarations about individual rights, which were given increasing prominence beginning in the 1960s, have propelled this principle to its dominant position today as the most influential principle of medical ethics.

The fourth principle, justice, differs from the first three in that it raises our sights from the individual patient to the needs of other individuals and/or of society. It has been born of necessity by the high cost of medical care and the scarcity of some resources. Secularists often combine the principles of justice and autonomy into a concept of citizenship and thus maintain that clinicians and patients have a responsibility to society and/or to nature for how resources are used.

There are other well-accepted concepts in medicine such as telling the truth (veracity), confidentiality, fidelity, and respect for persons. Many ethicists believe that these are subsumed under one or more of the "big four" and do not deserve the status of principles of medical ethics.

To summarize, secularists use these four principles to guide their medical ethics: doing good for patients (beneficence); "first of all, do no harm" (non-maleficence); self-determination (autonomy); responsibility to society and/or nature (justice).

Christians operate under the influence of principles as well, both in their personal lives and in the area of medical decision making. Many of these principles are comparable to and/or compatible with the secular principles listed above. Others are distinctive and not easily understood by the secularist, primarily because these principles arise either from biblical example or biblical revelation.

Christians, for example, also embrace the principles of doing good and not doing harm. For them, however, these principles include telling the truth and compassion, an inner motivation, which is implicit in the life of Jesus and is also explicitly taught in Scripture, as, for example, in the story of the good Samaritan.[2]

It is, however, over the matter of human autonomy that Christians and secularists have the greatest divergence of understanding. Christians believe that God created individuals in his image and has given individuals freedom to make decisions. Although he has given us dominion over nature, we are accountable to our Maker for the way we use our bodies, our talents, and our resources. Thus our autonomy is limited by the sovereignty of God, our Creator.

Christians believe the principle of justice requires charity and service in our daily lives as well as in the practice of medicine. The concept of justice as protection of the weak can be traced to the ancient Hebrew prophets and early Christian writers. In addition to earthly justice, Christians have a concept of divine justice tempered by God's mercy and grace. His justice was served by his placing our punishment on his Son. This gives the Christian an eternal hope, a perspective which is lacking from most non-Christian worldviews.

The Christian's foundational principle, the sanctity of life, is not stated explicitly in any one verse of Scripture but is clearly taught by precept throughout. For centuries this was also an integral part of the philosophy of medicine. Modern medical ethicists believe this principle has been replaced by "respect for persons" and is covered by the primary principle of doing good. Many Christians believe that this hallowed teaching has been, and continues to be, assaulted in modern thinking about abortion, suicide, euthanasia, and other life/death matters.

Beyond these principles, the Christian teaching that there may sometimes be value in suffering is completely foreign to the anthropocentric secular ethicist.

For the sake of comparison and review, let's set the secular and Christian approaches side by side.

These Perspectives Applied to Voluntary Sterilization

The secular assessment of voluntary sterilization is fairly straightforward. Since the primary concern of individuals with this perspective is protection of the individual, it is not surprising that the issues discussed in relation to sterilization are person centered. This is clearly followed in medical practice as well.

The medical profession rarely has addressed the ethics of sterilization. The American Medical Association's Council on Ethical and Judicial Affairs has produced no statement on sterilization and refers to it only briefly in its statement on genetic counseling. The American College of Obstetricians and Gynecologists in its 1989 opinion on "Ethical Considerations in Sterilization" emphasizes adequately informed consent, freedom of individual choice, privacy, protection of the vulnerable from coercion, physician competence, and freedom of conscience for the physician.[3] It adds that "the physician should encourage the patient to include appropriate persons in the counseling process."

Secularist	Christian
Human-centered Worldview	*God-centered Worldview*
•doing good for patients (beneficence), including respect for persons*	•involves compassion, following biblical precepts and Jesus' example
•avoiding harm (non-maleficence)	•includes truthfulness
•responsibility to society and/or nature (justice)	•involves charity and service and is founded on divine justice, which is tempered by God's mercy and grace

Conflicting Principles

•self-determination (autonomy)	•choices limited by the sovereignty of God, the Creator and according to the guidance of his Word
•respect for persons* has replaced sanctity of life	•sanctity of human life, sacred because it bears the image of God

Unique Principles

	•suffering can have a purpose, such as a person's correction, development, or the glory of God
	•eternity exists, which provides a sense of direction, purpose, hope, and even joy in the face of great adversity

*Note: Many people in defining persons, include only those who have self-awareness or the ability to relate to others.

It is generally accepted in secular thinking that a competent patient may choose to limit permanently his or her reproductive capacity for reasons of quantity control or quality control. Quantity control means it is acceptable to limit the number of children for reasons of physical health, socioeconomics, or personal convenience. Or patients may choose quantity control sterilization to limit their family size (or even choose to remain childless) to assure or maintain their personal quality of life.

Patients may also choose sterilization to avoid producing children with undesirable genetic characteristics (quality control). In other words, there are no secular right or wrong answers for voluntary sterilization as long as all statutory requirements such as informed consent, age, waiting periods, spousal consent, and second medical opinions have been met.[4]

By contrast, Christian perspectives on voluntary sterilization vary widely. The Roman Catholic Church has strongly adhered to a tradition which interprets as a procreation mandate Genesis 1:28: "God blessed them and said to them, 'Be fruitful and increase in number; fill the earth and subdue it.'"

The official church teaching, clearly articulated by Pope Paul IV in 1968, is that direct sterilization is intrinsically evil because of "the inseparable connection, willed by God and unable to be broken by man on his own initiative, between the two meanings of the conjugal act: the unitive meaning and the procreative meaning."[5]

Many Roman Catholic medical ethics writers have addressed sterilization. While there is general support for the official church teaching, some Catholic theologians do venture the opinion that although sterilization is a physical evil it does not constitute a moral evil "if there are correspondingly serious reasons for its performance."[6]

In commenting on the Roman Catholic position, J. T. Noonan points out that the church traditionally has encouraged married couples to procreate and educate children in the faith; that is, large families were not the primary goal, but it was necessary to raise children in the Roman Catholic tradition.[7]

In spite of clear and unwavering church teaching, however, the practice of a majority of Catholic couples is much less strict than official church position. A significant percentage use contraception or sterilization to limit their family size.

The vast majority of modern Protestant ethicists, on the other hand, believe that procreative decisions are personal decisions to be made by a couple using the principle of stewardship, which encompasses an individual's responsibility to use his or her time, talents, and resources in the service of God and for the benefit of humankind. This may be based either on the belief that stewardship outweighs those Scriptures which encourage procreation, or the interpretation that the procreation "mandate" is a blessing rather than a mandate. For example, a couple may decide that they will have only one or two children because the wife has chronic health problems that make it impossible for her to care for more children. Or another couple might believe that their income would allow them to provide an adequate education for three or four children, but would be spread too thin if they had more.

Either way, most Protestant ethicists approach sterilization very much like secular ethicists. Today most Protestant Christians have eagerly adopted contraceptive methods, including sterilization, as a means to limit their reproductive capability and capacity.

But this acceptance of sterilization is relatively new in Protestant thought and tradition. The Anglicans were the first Protestant group (1930) to break with the longstanding prohibition of contraception and sterilization because such matters were not only personal in nature, but also involved a significant social dimension (i.e. they had an impact on spouse, family, and society, as well as the individual).[8]

In view of this new freedom they encouraged reflection about the seriousness of the decision, they cautioned members about the importance of the methods chosen, and they condemned limitation of family size "from motives of selfishness, luxury, or mere convenience."[9]

Other faith traditions made the transition from prohibition to permission in the 1950s and 1960s. For example, the Reformed tradition suggested that couples give serious reflection to their reproductive decisions but also admonished thankful celebration if they are surprised by a gift of life.[10] In their view, voluntary childlessness for career advancement or economic inadequacy is not justified. However, the issue of family size was not addressed.

The Lutheran tradition also had a history of legalistic prohibition of contraception and sterilization, but in recent decades this has evolved into an almost universal acceptance of family planning.[11]

Similarly, the Methodist tradition has evolved from prohibition to the current stance that each couple has the right and the duty to prayerfully and responsibly control conception according to their circumstances.[12]

The National Council of the Churches of Christ in the USA, representing twenty-five denominations and thirty-seven million parishioners, adopted a position statement on contraception and sterilization in 1961, "Couples are free to use the gifts of science for conscientious family limitations. . . . Periodic continence (the rhythm method) is suitable for some couples, but is not inherently superior from a moral point of view. The general Protestant conviction is that motives, rather than methods, form the primary moral issue."[13] This points out what may be the major difference between Protestant and Roman Catholic thought on this issue. For Protestants, one's view on this is a conviction. The Catholic church sees the matter as one involving scriptural principles.

Many non-Catholic Christian authors have written books on medical ethics. Some do not address sterilization as an issue. Others decry involuntary sterilization for eugenic reasons. Several support the right of physicians to refuse to participate in sterilization based on their own conscience, but do not otherwise address the ethical issues of sterilization. Some find that although sterilization is not prohibited in Scripture, a decision for voluntary sterilization is a very weighty one and should not be made lightly. Still others consider the statement in Genesis 1:28 to be more of a blessing with historical particularity than a universal command; therefore, voluntary sterilization is acceptable.

The casualness with which many Christians have accepted sterilization is capsulized in the *Encyclopedia of Biblical & Christian Ethics* when it states, "Voluntary sterilization is indicated for socioeconomic, genetic, therapeutic, and personal reasons."[14]

Recently some conservative Christian individuals and congregations have rediscovered or reemphasized the procreation mandate. According to a 1991 *Christianity Today* Institute addressing birth control, "In some home-schooling and other countercultural circles, the notion that family planning is resisting God's sovereignty has taken root."[15] One writer in the Institute considered this a legalistic approach with a "mistaken notion of God's providence."[16]

Christian medical professional organizations have been remarkably permissive or totally silent on the issue of sterilization.

In August 1968, the Christian Medical Society (now, Christian Medical & Dental Society) and *Christianity Today* cosponsored "a Protestant Symposium on the Control of Human Reproduction." This was held soon after the discovery of new methods of contraception, in the midst of the "sexual revolution," at the beginning of public discussion about abortion, and shortly after the publication of *Humanae Vitae,* by Pope Paul IV. It represented "an effort by evangelical leaders to stay abreast of current developments and to appraise them from an authentically biblical point of view."[17] The multiple papers presented at the symposium clearly offered a permissive approach to voluntary sterilization for medical (including psychiatric), genetic, social, and personal reasons.

The Christian Medical & Dental Society (U.S.), which now has more than nine thousand Christian physicians and dentists and medical and dental student members, has formal written opinions on more than twenty issues in medical ethics. However, it has not addressed sterilization as an issue, nor is it mentioned in its statements on human sexuality, in vitro fertilization, or reproductive technology. Likewise, neither the CMDS of Canada nor the Christian Medical Fellowship in Great Britain has formulated a Christian ethical approach to sterilization.

In conclusion, secular medical ethics supports an individual's or couple's right to voluntary sterilization based on the principle of autonomy. Although Christians were fairly uniformly opposed to sterilization until fifty years ago, only the Roman Catholic church and a small minority of conservative Protestant Christians continue in this absolute opposition. Most Protestants allow voluntary sterilization for medical, genetic, socioeconomic, or personal reasons, using stewardship as the guiding principle. Some individuals and groups express concern about the casual acceptance of this option and encourage thoughtful and prayerful consideration before making this major decision. Others limit acceptable indications to nonselfish reasons. Most would consider motivations such as career advancement, personal economics, and freedom to travel or enjoy other pursuits to be "selfish" (i.e. self-centered, concerned primarily with one's own needs or desires). Most would also condone decisions made because of the poor health of the mother, total family economic pressures, or great potential for severe genetic defects. However, it is easy to see that there may be considerable overlap in these issues.

Which brings me back to Walter and Darcy. Let's suppose that they have sought my advice as a Christian clinical ethicist.

I might say, "The fact that you have asked for my opinion as a fellow believer indicates that you have decided that faith may have some bearing on what is acceptable in your case. I agree. And I believe it is in your best interests to study this question thoroughly until you can defend whatever decision you reach.

"In some ways, faith makes decisions such as this one more difficult. While secular ethics allow you to do whatever you want to do, faith requires you to subject your desires to the will of a higher authority, namely God. In this case, discerning his will is not easy because the Bible really doesn't directly address voluntary sterilization.

"That doesn't mean, however, that God is not concerned. It's similar to other issues, such as abortion, or euthanasia, or pulling the plug when someone is terminally ill. You have to search Scripture to find specific texts, principles, or examples that serve as an indicator of what God's perspective might be.

"In terms of voluntary sterilization, many Christians believe the command that God gave to Adam and Eve, to be fruitful and multiply, is still valid today. If you were to pursue sterilization before deciding what this command might mean for you personally, you might have severe regrets later.

"Or, to cite one more example, the Bible is quite consistent in describing children as a blessing from God. You seem sure that you don't want to have any. I respect your perspective, but suggest that you reconsider rejecting any blessing from the Lord. Further, you might ponder whether or not part of his plan for reaching the world with the good news is through the influence of Christian families. If this is true, perhaps you could view parenthood differently.

"Finally, there is the question of motives, which is perhaps the most difficult to resolve. Only you can know why you want to avoid having children. If the sole reason is to pursue your careers unhindered, I would have to say that I understand, as a professional person, how difficult it might be to try to start over after taking time out to raise a family. I would also say that in more than twenty years of family practice, I have seldom had a patient lament having put a career on hold for this purpose. Usually, the satisfaction and joys of parenthood far outweigh what has been lost. And I've never had any successful career person say how glad they were, on reaching middle age, that they had remained childless.

"As far as medical ethics goes, the secular approach leaves it entirely up to you. Christian medical ethics, however, would encourage you to delay sterilization until you have engaged in a thoughtful and thorough study of relevant verses, sought spiritual counsel, and prayed about it to the point where you are fully convinced that your decision will honor and please God. Once you have reached that point, I would be glad to discuss this matter with you again."

For Reflection or Discussion

Role play Darcy and Walter's discussion of their meeting with the family doctor.

1. Doctor Orr states that a person's worldview has a major impact on issues in the arena of medical ethics. Review, and expand if you like, the main issues for Darcy and Walter and the doctor as they try to see their decision from both sides. List these issues under the headings "Human centered" (anthropocentric) and "Christian."

2. Review the list of specific principles of moral reasoning in this chapter and write whatever principles you believe apply in their proper column. (Remember that some principles are common to both decision-making processes.)

3. Following completion of this exercise, have Darcy and Walter decide what they want to do. In preparation for revisiting their doctor they must answer the question about the basis of their decision. Then have them role play their next discussion with the doctor.

4. As you reflect on this entire exercise and the interactions involved, can you explain in a sentence why decision making in the arena of medical ethics can be more complicated for believers than for secularists?

5. Apply this understanding to the following cases. After going through the above process, decide what for each couple would be ethically defensible decisions.

Bill and Lois are a newly married Christian couple who have recently learned that Bill has Huntington's disease, an untreatable severe degenerative disease of the brain which begins in young adulthood and slowly but inexorably leads to dementia and death in a few years. There is a 50 percent chance that each child they have will also be affected. Bill is considering a vasectomy both to prevent the birth of a child with this horrible future and also to prevent Lois from having to raise children as a single mother. They wonder if these are justifiable reasons for sterilization.

Debbie and Charles have been married for ten years and have both worked at low-paying jobs. They have been able to make ends meet and started a small savings plan for the education of their two children, ages five and seven. They are considering sterilization because they fear they will be unable to afford college expenses for more than two children. Debbie attends a very conservative church which has a policy prohibiting sterilization (though it allows temporary methods of pregnancy prevention). Charles attends with her on Christmas and Easter, but he is not a believer. He thinks the church's ideas on most things, including permanent sterilization, are too conservative.

Theologically Sound

John Jefferson Davis

Steve and Joan

Thirty-year-old Steve, who was raised as a Roman Catholic, meets twenty-eight-year-old Joan at a single adults' hayride sponsored by her church, the Crossway Community Church, an independent Protestant church. Over the next few months Steve becomes "born again." He and Joan grow closer and then, to the delight of the group, announce their engagement. During premarital counseling, required of all couples who desire marriage in this church, the pastor discovers that Steve, to facilitate his rather profligate earlier lifestyle, had a vasectomy when he was twenty-five. Until he met Joan and experienced a renewal of his faith, marriage was not part of Steve's life plan. Joan, who is a virgin, tells the pastor she knows about the vasectomy, but still wants to marry Steve. The pastor says he will perform their marriage on the condition that Steve have surgery to reverse his vasectomy, because, in the pastor's words, "The primary purpose of Christian marriage is to raise up children for the Lord's army." Once this position becomes known in the singles group, after Joan mentions to her best friend that Steve can't afford the operation, the issue becomes quite divisive.

This hypothetical but not unlikely case illustrates the difficulty of the practical application of principles of Christian ethics to the question of voluntary sterilization, especially within independent Protestant churches. When Steve and Joan's pastor took his position, his authority derived mostly from his personal interpretation of relevant biblical ethics as pastor of that particular local body. Should the couple seek a second opinion from another local pastor, they might hear a completely different position. Additionally, the singles group's reaction illustrates the problem of enforcement when it comes to such a personal question. Perhaps this is why in Protestant circles and in Protestant writings the question of voluntary sterilization is seldom addressed in public. It is usually left entirely to the individuals involved. By contrast, the Roman Catholics have a long history of teachings related to this matter.

(The case study and introductory comments are mine. D. B. B.)

Roman Catholic Positions

As early as the First Council of Nicaea in A.D. 325 the Roman Catholic Church addressed issues that were at best indirectly related to the modern issue of contraceptive sterilization. In a canon, or declaration of church law, concerning those "who make themselves eunuchs and others who suffer the same loss at the hands of others," the council ruled that those who had been castrated for medical reasons or who had been castrated by persecuting barbarians could still remain members of the clergy. Those, however, who in good health had voluntarily chosen castration (perhaps like Father Origen, as an extreme form of ascetical piety) should be suspended from the ministry.[1]

Already in the fourth century, the Roman Catholic tradition was viewing any deliberate destruction of the person's procreative power as a form of mutilation of the body that was not justifiable except in unusual cases of medical necessity.

It was only during the latter part of the nineteenth century, however, subsequent to the development of modern surgical techniques of tubal ligation and vasectomy, that the church's teaching on elective contraceptive sterilization became crystallized.

In 1895 the Vatican declared that no active or passive procedure performed for the express purpose of sterilizing a woman was permissible. In his 1930 encyclical on Christian marriage, Pope Pius XI condemned eugenic sterilization. In 1940 the Vatican declared that direct sterilization, temporary or permanent, whether of a man or a woman, was contrary to the law of nature. This general position was reaffirmed by Pius XII in 1951 and 1958, and by Paul VI in 1964.[2]

The problem of sterilization has received extensive attention from Roman Catholic ethicists during this century. In his 1959 discussion, Thomas J. O'Donnell, S. J., in keeping with the teaching of the magisterium, noted that directly intended contraceptive sterilization is not permitted. The generative organs exist not merely for the good of the individual but for the good of the species. Contraceptive sterilization is beyond the scope of man's proper dominion over his own body.[3] However, he explained, when a diseased organ, as part of the body, becomes destructive of the good of the whole body, as in the case of a cancerous uterus,[4] the "principle of totality" justifies the surgical removal of the uterus, even in spite of the (unintended) sterilizing effect. Similarly, it may be morally justifiable to irradiate healthy ovaries in cases of malignant breast cancer, if it is likely that the resulting inhibition of hormonal activity would retard the spread of the cancer and possibly save the patient's life.[5]

In his 1967 discussion, Charles J. McFadden argues that the principle of totality obliges one to employ all reasonable means to preserve life and health. No vital organ or bodily function should be suppressed or removed unless such an action is directed toward "the cure or alleviation of some pathology presently existing in the body."[6] Our basic duty is to preserve the integrity of the body as much as is reasonably possible, he said.

However, McFadden added, in the cases of some pathologies it may be necessary to preserve the welfare of the whole person through the sacrifice of a part.[7] For example, prostate cancer is a very painful disease, the development and spread of which is fostered by the male androgens, principally supplied by the testes (testicles). Irradiation of the testes, or even surgical removal of the testes (orchidectomy) may be medically indicated. Such procedures would, of course, produce sterility, but would be morally justified to preserve the patient's life.

In their 1989 discussion, Benedict Ashley and Kevin O'Rourke employ the accepted distinction between direct and indirect sterilization. Rather than being a treatment for pathology, direct sterilization has contraception as its direct and primary purpose. When sterility results merely as a side effect of a medical procedure intended to treat a specific pathology, it is said to be indirect and can be justified by the principle of totality.[8] The authors cite a 1971 directive of the United States Catholic Conference to Catholic hospitals, which states that sterilizing procedures are permitted only when they are directed toward serious pathological conditions, contraception not being the intended purpose, and simpler treatments are not available. Therefore, orchidectomy would be permissible in cases of prostate cancer.

Some Roman Catholic ethicists have dissented from the church's official teachings on sterilization. Richard A. McCormick, for example, has questioned the assumption that direct sterilization would always constitute an unethical attack on the well-being of the person. In his view, a broader understanding of the principle of totality—including the total well-being of the person in all relationships and personal, economic, and spiritual circumstances—could justify an analysis in which the negative effect of loss of procreative ability was outweighed by positive effects of the procedure. According to McCormick, the loss of ability to procreate may not in every instance be an intrinsic evil which harms the moral well-being of the person.[9]

Protestant Positions

The Church of England was one of the first of the Protestant bodies to take a public position on the question of sterilization. The Anglican leaders at the 1958 Lambeth Conference agreed that sterilization could be justified in cases of imperative medical necessity, such as hysterectomy in the case of uterine cancer.[10] However, in the case of voluntary contraceptive sterilization, the generally irreversible nature of such procedures, the possible psychological impact on both spouses, the violation of the human body as a divine trust, and the perhaps unforeseen long-term consequences, are factors that should be weighed most seriously.[11] Nevertheless, the conference did conclude that such procedures could be morally acceptable.

Dietrich Bonhoeffer, a German Lutheran pastor and theologian, was executed in 1945 at age thirty-nine in a Nazi concentration camp. His writings in the area of Christian ethics were posthumously edited by his friend Eberhard Bethge and published under the title *Ethics*.

Bonhoeffer addressed the issue of sterilization both in its voluntary and state-mandated forms. He asserted that the human body possesses "an inherent right of inviolability. Neither I nor the state can lay claim to an absolute right of free disposal over the bodily members that have been given to me by God."[12]

Bonhoeffer held that in cases of medical necessity to preserve the patient's life, surgical sterilization is permissible as the lesser of two evils. However, in cases where self-control is possible, voluntary sterilization is not permissible. Such procedures would be unwarranted infringements on the "natural right of reproduction," in Bonhoeffer's view.[13]

Another German Lutheran theologian, Helmut Thielicke, writing in 1964, notes that the moral issues relating to sterilization are not "fundamentally different" from those of contraception, with the exception of the question of permanence or irreversibility. Thielicke has no explicit discussion of voluntary sterilization.

The liberal Protestant ethicist Joseph Fletcher devoted one chapter in his book *Morals and Medicine* (1954) to the question of sterilization. In contrast to Roman Catholic approaches stressing "integrity of the body," Fletcher argued that the emphasis should be on the "integrity of the personality."[14] (Fletcher later became the exponent of situation ethics.)

His view was that moral responsibility requires that choices regarding sterilization be "personal decisions rather than natural necessities."[15] When there are good and sufficient reasons to eliminate the possibility of reproduction to "fulfill the obligations of love," we are ethically justified in doing so, he claimed. He asserted a right to choose preventive sterilization in the face of anticipated birth defects; such a choice would save "potentially defective children from being thrown into a life of misery and futility."[16]

Fletcher explicitly argues for the ethical justifiability of *therapeutic and preventive* sterilization, but the logic of his argument would seem to implicitly justify *elective* or *voluntary, contraceptive* sterilization as well.

Evangelical Protestants have also given attention to the issue of sterilization. A 1968 symposium on "The Control of Human Reproduction" was sponsored by the Christian Medical Society (now the Christian Medical & Dental Society) in cooperation with the editors of *Christianity Today* magazine. Several of the papers presented at the symposium dealt in at least a preliminary way with sterilization and were included in the volume published in 1969 under the title *Birth Control and the Christian*.

In general, their perspective was very permissive. For example, the summary Affirmation statement of the symposium says: "We live in a world pervaded by evil. Human relationships are distorted; unwanted children are born . . . genetic defects are not uncommon and harmful social conditions abound. Therefore, it is the duty of Christians to be compassionate to individuals and to seek responsibly to mitigate the effects of evil when possible, in accordance with the . . . principles (of sanctity of family life and the responsibility, fulfillment, self-discipline and divine grace in sexual relationship).

"When principles conflict," the statement adds, "the preservation of fetal life or the integrity of the human body may have to be abandoned in order to maintain full and secure family life."[17]

Writing in a pre-1973, pre-*Roe v. Wade* moral climate, prior to the legalization of abortion in the United States, many of the contributors to this 1969 volume expressed perspectives on abortion and related issues significantly different from the prevailing climate of opinion in evangelical circles today.

British evangelical author J. N. D. Anderson addressed issues of birth control and sterilization in his book *Issues of Life and Death* (1976). Anderson noted that while there is no direct prohibition of sterilization in the Bible, the Scriptures do teach that man is a created being who does not have an unlimited right to dispose of himself as he wishes. Therefore, the human body may not be treated arbitrarily or mutilated except where necessary.[18]

As to what constitutes necessity[19] in relation to voluntary sterilization, Anderson said, the medical advisor should interpret the doctrine of necessity in a realistic way in relation to the terms of the particular case.[20]

In his book on medical ethics, *Making Biblical Decisions* (1989), Christian physician Franklin E. Payne, Jr. agreed with Helmut Thielicke that "the decision [to be sterilized] is correspondingly more momentous, but not fundamentally different [from contraception in general]."[21] However, he asserted that for believers the procreation of children is the norm and sterilization is the exception.

Payne recommended that sterilization should not be considered unless the couple has had three or more children (because for two individuals to "multiply" requires three) or is facing some serious impediments to having a larger family.[22] Furthermore, before making any such choice, one should seriously consider the possibility that one could lose a spouse, remarry, or desire additional children during the fertile years.[23]

In *Ethics For a Brave New World* (1993), evangelical scholars John and Paul Feinberg noted that the modern problem of elective surgical sterilization is not really addressed in Scripture.

Biblical texts such as Deuteronomy 23:1, Matthew 19:10–12, Acts 8, which refer to eunuchs are, in the Feinbergs' view, at best only tangentially related to the discussion at hand. They also have serious doubts as to whether the statement of Genesis 1:28 to fill the earth is universally applicable in ways that are relevant to the issue of sterilization.

Without explicitly referring to the Roman Catholic principle of totality, the authors believe that sterilization could be medically advisable in cases where a history of difficult pregnancies and deliveries indicates that further childbearing could endanger the woman's health.[24]

The Feinbergs observe that Christians should affirm "the great joy, privilege and blessing from God of parenting," and include such considerations in decisions concerning number of children.[25] However, they conclude that no scriptural or logical considerations rule out voluntary sterilization.[26]

Review of Pertinent Bible Texts

The text in Deuteronomy 23:1, "No one who has been emasculated by crushing or cutting may enter the assembly of the LORD," is probably not intended to bar from the community those whose state of emasculation was due to accident or illness.[27] The reference may, in fact, be to individuals for whom castration involves ritual dedication to the service of pagan gods or goddesses.[28] Saggs notes that in Mesopotamian religion eunuchs seemed to have dressed in female clothing, in cultic acts related to the fertility goddess Ishtar. In the Mishnah are rabbinic discussions of Deuteronomy 23:1 in relation to the right to participate in the eating of the heave-offering and the contracting of levirate marriages.

Taken in its context, therefore, this text has little relevance to the modern question of elective sterilization.

In Matthew 19:12 Jesus refers to those who have made themselves eunuchs for the sake of the kingdom of heaven. These "eunuchs" may be those disciples of Jesus who, after divorcing their wives for immorality, voluntarily live in a state of singleness and do not remarry.[29] In the context of the Jewish culture with its clear insistence on marriage, the words of Jesus "urge full acceptance of such men in the Christian brotherhood."[30] W. C. Allen takes the text to refer to such instances of the renunciation of marriage as "the Essenes, or John the Baptist, or some among his disciples." So understood, the text would not bear directly on the question of elective surgical sterilization.

Clearly relevant to the discussion is the "cultural mandate" of the first chapter of Genesis: "God blessed them and said to them, 'Be fruitful and increase in number; fill the earth and subdue it'" (Genesis 1:28). Some commentators have raised the question as to whether Gen. 1:28 is to be understood as a *blessing* on procreation or a *command* to procreate. Both senses are possible readings of the Hebrew imperatival verb. For an imperative used in blessing, see Genesis 24:60; Exodus 4:18; Deuteronomy 33:18.[31]

"This command," notes Gordon Wenham, "carries with it an implicit promise that God will enable man to fulfill it."[32] In Wenham's view, Genesis 1:28 is a clear statement of the purpose of marriage. Positively, it is for the procreation of children; negatively it is a rejection of the ancient pagan fertility cults.[33] "God desires his people to be fruitful," he states.[34]

Other biblical texts that support procreation as the purpose of marriage are the following:

> Large families are seen as an important dimension of God's blessing on Abraham and his descendants (Gen. 13:16; 15:5; 17:5, 6; 22:17; 28:13, 14).
> God continues to make his covenant people fruitful in childbearing even under conditions of oppression in Egypt (Exod. 1:12, 20, 21).
> The psalmists celebrate large families as a blessing from God (Ps. 127:3–5; 128:1–4).

The prophet Malachi, writing to the people of Israel after the exile, reminds them that the Lord desires "godly offspring" (Mal. 2:15).

The apostle Paul exhorts the younger widows in Ephesus to remarry and to bear children (1 Tim. 5:14). This admonition may have been directed against an incipient form of gnostic teaching that devalued marriage, sexuality, and childbearing. The text assumes that the "cultural mandate" of Genesis 1:28 is still valid in the New Testament age.

The principles of Christian care for the body articulated by the apostle in 1 Corinthians 6:19, 20 are pertinent to the present discussion: "Do you not know that your body is a temple of the Holy Spirit, who is in you, whom you have received from God? You are not your own; you were bought at a price. Therefore honor God with your body."

The apostle's point is that the believer does not have the right to exercise unlimited dominion over his or her body but should view the body as a trust from the Lord, to be cared for in ways that are glorifying to God.

Any surgical operation—such as sterilization—is not merely a personal "choice," but a decision that needs to be seen within a biblical framework of stewardship of the human body.

Given the fact that our human bodies are a trust from God, and in light of the positive valuation placed on human procreative powers and large families in the Old Testament, these powers should not be rejected or surgically destroyed without compelling justification.

Conclusion

Based on these relevant biblical texts and principles, and in light of the various traditions and ethical perspectives examined in this chapter, my view is that surgical sterilization is not justifiable as a matter of personal convenience; rather, it is only justifiable in cases of serious personal hardship or where additional pregnancies pose substantial threats to the life or health of the mother or to the welfare of the family unit.

For example, let's suppose Dick, who is a business executive, and Jane, who is a neonatologist in an academic setting, have no children. They have concluded that sterilization is a question of personal preference, since the Bible does not address it directly.

Dick wants a vasectomy because he honestly doesn't like children. Also, he is afraid that becoming a father might divert resources he'd rather accumulate. Beyond that, fatherhood might prevent his enjoying some of his favorite, rather expensive, recreational pursuits. In my opinion, Dick's sterilization would not be justifiable, because his motives are primarily selfish.

Jane also wants no children because, if she were to take even a few years off to start a family, she might put her academic appointment at risk. This motivation, in my view, is more reasonable, but in light of the biblical texts and principles we've examined, it would not be justifiable, since even if Jane were to lose some ground on her contemporaries, the welfare of the family unit would not be substantially threatened.

On the other hand, if Jane had a medical condition in which pregnancy might pose a significant threat to her life or health, or if this couple were going permanently to a mission field where having young children might put the children, themselves, or the larger family unit, at risk, this decision to remain childless might be more justifiable.

In a society where surgical sterilization has become common, American Christians in particular need to be challenged anew by the biblical witness to the blessings of children, and the scriptural mandate to "be fruitful and multiply."

This brings up the practical question of how many children should Christian couples try to have, if they take this mandate seriously? Demographically speaking, the number must be more than two. Since not all children survive to adulthood, the replacement rate necessary to simply maintain our population at its current level is 2.12 children per woman. Therefore, couples who believe they should try to "be fruitful," must produce at least one child. If they want to "multiply," they will aim at having (through procreation or adoption) at least three children.

Christian couples who have three or more children, view them as a gift from God, and raise them in the nurture and instruction of the Lord, are participating in one of the greatest processes and privileges of life. In general, they will not see having children as a great personal sacrifice driven by what others might label an unfortunate sense of obligation arising from poor biblical exegesis. Instead, they will joyfully embrace parenthood as an opportunity to make a significant contribution not only to the kingdom of God, but also to the need for godly character and future leadership in our nation and around the world.

For Reflection or Discussion

1. What is your response to the dilemma faced by Steve and Joan?

   ___ What dilemma? This hypothetical case could never happen.

   ___ Steve created the problem for the wrong reasons. He should get it fixed if he can.

   ___ Joan loves Steve the way he is. The pastor is intruding.

   ___ Joan is making a mistake, which the pastor is trying to help her avoid.

   ___ The singles group should take a collection to pay for Steve's surgery.

   ___ If Steve is a "new creation" in Christ, perhaps his mistakes are covered by the grace of God.

   ___ Sterilization should never be coerced.

   ___ Other

2. Discuss the Roman Catholic position with regard to voluntary sterilization.

___ I had no idea that it could be traced back so far.

___ The position has been the most consistent and clear of any available.

___ It is out of touch with the realities of family life.

___ I wish it was as founded in biblical exegesis as in tradition.

___ It may be the most reliable, but I can't afford to put it into practice.

___ Other

3. Review and evaluate the helpfulness of these Protestant perspectives reviewed in this chapter:

   ___ Church of England's Lambeth Conference
   ___ Bonhoeffer
   ___ Fletcher
   ___ Anderson
   ___ Payne
   ___ Feinbergs

4. Select the biblical text or principle mentioned in this chapter that is the most compelling to you personally. Restate in one sentence its key precept. Then try to express this truth's practical application to your own life, if any.

5. Evaluate and discuss Davis's conclusion:

   "My view is that surgical sterilization is not justifiable as a matter of personal convenience; rather, it is justifiable only in cases of serious personal hardship or where additional pregnancies pose substantial threats to the life or health of the mother or to the welfare of the family unit.

   "In a society where surgical sterilization has become common, American Christians in particular need to be challenged anew by the biblical witness to the blessings of chil-

dren (Ps. 127, 128) and the scriptural mandate to 'be fruitful and multiply.'"

6. Using this statement as a guide and the scriptural refer-
   ences as a foundation, try to develop a rough draft for a
   position paper on this subject. You will come back to this
   again, so don't try to perfect it this time around.

Morally
Acceptable

David B. Biebel

Polly and Peter

With her husband Peter's full agreement, Polly had her tubes tied when she was thirty-five, just minutes after the birth of the couple's third child. In asking the doctor to do this, Polly and Peter had the support of their friends, family, and pastor, whom they consulted ahead of time. For the next three years they lived relatively peacefully.

Then Peter's employer transferred him to another city, where the family searched for a church. The closest they could come to the one they had left was a somewhat more conservative but friendly enough group that was full of young families, most of them larger than theirs. One Sunday morning, an itinerant evangelist preached a very convincing and convicting sermon about how Christians should not cut off generations of future believers by getting sterilized. Before the service ended, Peter and Polly were standing before the altar repenting of their "sin."

The problem with some medically informed, ethically defensible, theologically sound decisions is that they may be morally acceptable to one individual or group and morally unacceptable, or sinful, to another individual or group. The result is that what once seemed to be a morally acceptable decision, in retrospect appears to be wrong.

Some activities which seem perfectly okay to some Christians may cause great alarm to others. Since this is true of minor behavioral issues such as modes of dress or attending the theater, it should not surprise us to find a major difference of opinion among sincere, Bible-believing, evangelical Christians about the much more significant matter of voluntary sterilization.

The main unresolved question of sterilization is moral in nature. The word *moral* comes from the word *mores* (pronounced mor-ays), "the fundamental moral beliefs of a social group." Mores either overtly or subtly influence personal decisions about sterilization, as they do any other decision. Since we all live in social networks—including family, church, community, nation—we have been exposed to many systems of morality over time. These beliefs influence our attitudes and actions more than we usually realize.

For example, if we lived in an overpopulated nation where the government had decreed that for the good of the state couples should have no more than one child, we might feel guilty violating this standard by having, say, two children. By contrast, we might deem ourselves good citizens for seeking sterilization immediately after our first child was born. These guilty feelings and good evaluations would be rooted primarily in the group's definition of morality in relation to childbearing.

A similar result can come from more subtle coercion. In the late 1960s, when my wife and I were married, the Zero Population Growth (ZPG) movement made it seem like a moral imperative that enlightened couples do their part to reduce the rate of the world's population explosion by limiting their family size. I have no idea how many of our contemporaries were sterilized because of this sense of duty, but even now there appears to be a subtle sense of disapproval in the church and society at large when couples choose to have large families. One who sees a pregnant woman struggling to control four preschoolers in the grocery store, all of whom call her Mommy, may be tempted to wonder, *Hasn't she ever heard of birth control?*

While most people's moral systems are greatly influenced by various social groups, Christians must be careful not to let their moral system, which guides their attitudes, beliefs, and actions, be defined by anything other than Scripture.

However, many churchgoing Christians today have not had enough broad exposure to Scripture or their church's interpretation to know what God has said that might directly or indirectly relate to the issue they are considering. Their approach to sterilization might be to declare that God isn't much concerned about this matter because their concordance does not list the subject.

Where There Is No "Vision"

This whole issue of voluntary sterilization would be much easier if the Bible said somewhere that it is either acceptable or unacceptable to God. But it doesn't. You can't find this matter either prescribed ("you should do it") or proscribed ("you shouldn't do it") in the biblical text. In other words, in relation to this topic, there is no "vision," or word from God through one of his prophets.

For some, this silence implies total freedom of choice, within limitations established by their conscience. This approach is risky if my own experience with guidance by conscience goes, because I may go ahead and do what is right in my eyes, but without some guidance from the Lord, I can't trust myself to do what is right in his eyes. I will often choose to do what is expedient rather than what is edifying, to me or others. As Proverbs 14:12 says, "There is a way that seems right to a man, but in the end it leads to death." The prophet Jeremiah warned that "The heart is deceitful above all things and beyond cure. Who can understand it?" (Jer. 17:9).

Only God understands the deceitfulness of the human heart, and only he can do something to cure that, through faith in Christ, which produces a renewal of spirit, heart, and mind, and allows a human being to discern, choose, and do the will of God. This becomes more of a spiritual habit as we grow in faith and understanding of not only what the Bible says about a specific topic, but also which examples or principles in its pages may apply to the debatable issue at hand.

For instance, the Bible nowhere expressly forbids slavery, or abortion, or many other despicable things that have been done or are currently being done "with a clear conscience" by people calling themselves Christians. The case against these things must be developed on the basis of broader principles derived from relevant examples or texts. When this approach is applied to voluntary sterilization, I believe that we can find enough data to build a solid foundation for our beliefs and practice in this area.

Earlier in this book, Youngberg and Davis mentioned texts from both Old and New Testaments in which physical fruitfulness is exhorted: Genesis 1:28, 9:1; and Timothy 5:14. This is one of the primary purposes for marriage and is consistently viewed as a blessing in the Scriptures. Throughout the ages, God's plan for advancing his kingdom has included the physical fruitfulness of his people.

God's plan also includes his people's spiritual fruitfulness. Gen. 22:17–18 may have a spiritual meaning as well as physical in that the true children of Abraham, according to the apostle Paul, are those who share Abraham's faith (Rom. 4:16; Gal. 3:7). In John 15:1–8, Jesus speaks of his disciples bearing fruit to God's glory, an obviously spiritual analogy. However, this does not justify the position that since in this present age God wants to advance his kingdom through spiritual means, physical fruitfulness has diminished as part of his plan to fill the earth with the knowledge of himself.

Consistently throughout Scripture, barrenness is viewed as undesirable. (Involuntarily infertile modern couples need not interpret their inability to reproduce as a sign that God has withdrawn his blessing. Infertility is a growing problem today and the source of great pain to couples who face it, but it is beyond the scope of this book.) As Jesus was being led out of Jerusalem to be crucified, he said that in a difficult time that was coming (some think he was referring to a time of great tribulation), barrenness would be considered a blessing (Luke 23:29). Possibly he said it because children in such a situation would hinder the family unit's ability to escape their enemies, or perhaps because children in such times are very vulnerable and seeing them suffer is doubly traumatic for their parents. On this basis, it could be argued, couples ministering in dangerous situations, for instance in some places on the mission field, might choose not to have children. However, since many effective temporary forms of pregnancy prevention are available, it seems unwise to pursue sterilization, especially when the couple is still relatively young.

Beyond this reference, however, the Bible contains no passage or principle presenting diminished reproductive capacity as either good or desirable. As far as Scripture is concerned, unless pregnancy would actually threaten the life of the wife, it is reasonable to infer that it is still normal for married believers to try to "be fruitful."

Psalm 127:3-5 says that "sons are a heritage from the LORD, children a reward from him. Like arrows in the hands of a warrior are sons born in one's youth. Blessed is the man whose quiver is full of them. They will not be put to shame when they contend with their enemies in the gate." Other Old Testament passages echo this positive regard for children. Jacob told Esau that his children were given to him by God (Gen. 33:5). Isaiah said, "Here am I, and the children the LORD has given me" (Isa. 8:18). By contrast, the secular individual says, "These are the children I have given myself."

On the basis of these texts, Christian couples who choose childlessness for reasons of selfishness, personal convenience, finances, or to pursue a career unhindered, are rejecting something God views as a heritage, a reward, a gift, or a blessing. To view something as a liability which the Lord holds in such positive esteem seems to be not very spiritually discerning.

However, the fact that children are a heritage, reward, gift, or blessing does not necessarily obligate Christian couples to produce as many children as possible. For the mere fact that a quiver full of children is a blessing suggests that anyone's "quiver" may be full. This might be because no more arrows will fit in. Or perhaps the quiver is so amply supplied that no more arrows are needed. The second meaning may be more in line with what the psalmist has in mind, since he is using a warfare analogy. Simply put, you don't want to get into battle and run out of ammunition before your enemy does. In a spiritual sense, believers are soldiers in the Lord's army, which is constantly contending with the forces of the enemy in the "gate" of the world for the minds and souls of people. Therefore, a case may be made that having a "quiver" full of children to launch against this enemy is still a blessing.

I hesitate to build too much practical theology on this text, but I do think a couple of valid points might be drawn from it. One is that having a full quiver is a good thing. Whether any couple's "quiver" is chock full or simply amply supplied will probably be defined by the couple according to their resources or purposes. Having said this, however, we add that even couples who believe they must do their part before God to "fill the earth" might at some point decide that they have filled their quiver.

For believers who think they are obligated to have as many children as possible, the key texts are Genesis 1:28 and 9:1. In trying to discern how these texts apply to Christians thousands of years later we should keep in mind that in both cases when the mandates were given the earth was "empty." Adam and Eve had not yet had any children. Noah and his sons and their wives had just emerged from the ark. Whether the earth is now full may be debatable, but it is certainly not still empty in the same sense that it was when the original commands were issued.

Beyond that, it is theologically risky to universalize a mandate with such obvious historical application unless it is repeated elsewhere in Scripture in a more general sense. Fruitfulness is still operative, yes, and children are still to be highly esteemed. Seeking to "fill the earth," however, may not be morally obligatory today.

But what about the phrase "increase in number"? This still may be operative if it is implied by "fruitfulness" or by Paul's exhortation that young widows should remarry and bear children.[1] If you believe that this part of the mandate is still valid, logic requires that you will try to have more than two offspring, for the reasons Dr. Davis explained.

At this point, let me summarize the practical biblical principles related to sterilization:

Fruitfulness is a primary purpose of marriage, a blessing from God, and one of his strategies for enlarging his kingdom. Therefore, Christian couples should try to have children. If they believe that God wants them to "increase in number," they will try to have more than two children.

Childlessness by choice should be the exception for believers, though it is acceptable in special circumstances. The command to "fill the earth" may not be binding today, since it was given in special circumstances and it is not repeated elsewhere in Scripture. Couples who believe this command is still morally obligatory, however, may still reach a point when they believe they have fulfilled their obligation by filling their "quiver."

Is Sterilization Acceptable?

This brings us to an important juncture in the process of defining a biblically based practical position about voluntary sterilization. The question is: If it is acceptable under some conditions to *temporarily* limit one's fertility, is it acceptable to *permanently* limit one's fertility through sterilization? For some people, these issues are identical, or so nearly identical, that nothing further need be said. Those who oppose temporary forms of pregnancy prevention will oppose sterilization. Those who allow temporary forms of pregnancy prevention will apply the same latitude to sterilization.

However, I believe that elective sterilization should be placed in a different category for several reasons. First, it requires surgery with its physical risks. Second, the long-term psychological and physical risks of sterilization are not known. Third, the motivation of people seeking sterilization may be different from those who practice temporary forms of pregnancy prevention, which renders elective sterilization different in form and substance from temporary pregnancy prevention.

The risks associated with tubal ligation for women are significant, but still less than those associated with pregnancy.

For men, the statistical incidence of physical complications of vasectomy is greater than complications for women. But none of the complications is life threatening. Although recent scientific studies found a possible statistical link between vasectomy and prostate cancer, initial data from ongoing studies predict no significant link will be shown.

The problem for patients is that percentages express themselves in the form of persons when you or someone you love is the exception. Before proceeding with sterilization, therefore, a couple should prayerfully discuss the possible complications one by one and ask themselves, "Is permanent prevention of pregnancy worth this risk?" Or, to ask it a different way, "If my spouse experienced this complication as a result of this surgery, would I ever forgive myself?"

Psychological Risks

Beyond the medical risks are psychological risks worth noting. Dr. McIlhaney mentioned some rare reactions that occur in sterilized women. Also, men may experience psychological reactions that they keep to themselves. Additionally, some people would argue that for women the psychological impact of unplanned pregnancy outweighs the physical risks. But to accept that argument you have to decide whether, within the context of the providence of God, *any* pregnancies can be unplanned.

Motivation

A third factor, and perhaps the most important one, that puts sterilization in a different moral category from temporary birth control is the motivation of the couple involved. Clearly, the Bible is not concerned with only actions or consequences. From the tenth commandment—You shall not covet—to the teachings of Jesus, the Scriptures emphasize that a person's thoughts and motives are what really drive his or her actions. Therefore, the only way to please God is not by always doing the right things (which you couldn't, even if you wanted to), or by doing more right things than wrong things (since there are no divine scales of justice), but to bring your thoughts and motives captive to the will of God.

The problem with motives is that very few of us know ourselves well enough, or are willing to face ourselves if we know ourselves well enough, to truly discern why we have done or might want to do something. This is why searching the Scriptures with an open heart and mind, allowing God's Spirit to show us not only his will but our true selves, is so important to this question. "For the word of God is living and active. Sharper than any double-edged sword, it penetrates even to dividing soul and spirit, joints and marrow; it judges the thoughts and attitudes of the heart" (Heb. 4:12).

Suppose, for example, that after the birth of our first child, I had gotten a vasectomy because I resented Jonathan's taking a lot of the time and attention my wife used to give to me. You would be right in questioning my motives.

Choosing to become a parent is choosing to give up many of your "rights" and a lot of your space during a good part of your most productive years in exchange for the joy of having God knock off a lot of your rough edges through your kids.

People get sterilized because they don't want to surrender these things. Some parents get sterilized because they figure they've surrendered enough. On the other hand, many parents embrace the inconvenience, adjust their expectations, and gladly welcome more children if God so blesses them. It's more than a matter of choice. It's a matter of the heart.

Quite commonly, couples who have several children realize, on the basis of their experience and consideration of their resources, that if they have any more children they may not be able to provide as well for the others, whether the provision be food, clothing, shelter, education, or nurture. This is stewardship, the management of resources for the benefit of others. From my perspective, it's hard to criticize these motives, since they are generated not so much by the personal desires of the parents as by their wish to take proper care of their children. For, as the apostle Paul said, "If anyone does not provide for his relatives, and especially for his immediate family, he has denied the faith and is worse than an unbeliever" (1 Tim. 5:8).

The only caution I would urge with this line of thinking is that in Western countries today "provision" is often "conspicuous consumption" in disguise. Nonetheless, I believe that conscientious Christian parents who have fulfilled the relevant biblical exhortations about fruitfulness may conclude with a pure heart before God that the stewardship of their resources and energy requires them to permanently limit their procreative capacity. This will be done out of love for God and their family.

When they choose to go ahead with this procedure, however, believers need to realize that the net effect is to take their reproductive capacity totally and permanently under their own control. Crossing this line is a matter of substance for believers who accept the biblical teaching that they are not their own but are God's (1 Cor. 6:19–20) and that he is the ultimate controller of their destinies (including their reproductive destinies). Some will not be able to cross this line in good conscience.

A Mutual Decision

None should be able to cross this line in good conscience unless they are acting in total harmony as a couple, for the Bible also teaches that "The wife's body does not belong to her alone but also to her husband. In the same way, the husband's body does not belong to him alone but also to his wife" (1 Cor. 7:4).

Stan had a vasectomy six years ago without his wife's agreement. In all this time, the two of them have not been able to talk about the subject. Like almost any stressor, sterilization for either spouse can exacerbate problems in their relationship that already exist, unless there is a settled, shared conviction that this is the right and best thing to do.

Even when there seems to be a settled, shared conviction, it is always best to check one last time before proceeding. A physician told me about a husband who came in seeking a vasectomy. His wife had just delivered twins following a very difficult pregnancy, complicated by her incompetent cervix (which often results in a premature delivery). One of the twins was hospitalized for some time.

"I asked Charlie what his wife's sentiments were," the doctor said. "Well, Ellie really thinks she might want to have a baby again," Charlie replied. "But her doctor in Boston said she shouldn't have any more." The doctor sent Charlie home to talk it over with Ellie.

Not long thereafter, the man came in a second time for an exam in preparation for the procedure itself. "We're together on it now," Charlie said. But this particular doctor does not do a sterilization until the third visit, even though this takes much more of his time and therefore costs him potential revenue from other patients.

On the third visit the wife came, too, to drive her husband home after the surgery. With everything prepared for the procedure, the doctor checked once more. He took the couple into an adjacent room. "A couple of visits ago Charlie mentioned you had some reservations about this," the doctor said.

"Oh, yeah," Ellie replied. "If I knew that I could go through a pregnancy and have a baby and everything would be all right, I'd sure like to have another baby."

"Well, did your doctor in Boston tell you you should never have another baby?" the doctor asked.

"Oh, no," she said.

Her husband looked at her and said, "I thought he did say that."

"No," she said, "he never did." Then she paused and looked at the doctor. "My mother and my sisters and a lot of other people say we shouldn't have any more children," she admitted.

Forty-five minutes later, after praying and counseling with the couple about their decision, the doctor said, "I can't in good conscience do the procedure today. If you want to find somebody else to do it, that is okay. But if you do, please do me the courtesy to notify me. I won't harbor any hard feelings, but I will pray for you as you ponder this some more."

Vasectomy is the most often canceled procedure in this country, probably because of issues like this, along with many men's natural aversion to having anything sharp in the vicinity of their reproductive parts.

Going Ahead

All things considered, however, a couple may with a totally clear conscience decide on sterilization if they can say in effect, "As God's servants and as good stewards of our procreative capacities we will seek to glorify him by raising up as godly offspring the quiver full of children he has already given us. To better provide for their physical, emotional, and spiritual needs, we believe it is morally acceptable in his sight to seek permanent sterilization."

In reaching the settled decision to either have sterilization or not, it seems prudent that the couple seek the godly input of trusted advisors which might include their parents, other relatives, their pastor, and their church (through the elders or a trusted circle of friends).

Ultimately, however, each couple's motives will be unique and known only to them and God, so there is no way for a third party to legitimately dictate a specific rule about sterilization that applies across the board. In summary, then, the following should have direct bearing on that decision:

Sterilization has both medical and psychological risks. A couple should pursue it only after intensive biblical and spiritual reflection aimed at discerning the thoughts and intentions of their own hearts. The procedure should only be performed if a couple shares the settled belief, perhaps reached with the assistance of trusted advisors, that under no circumstances would God want them to have another child.

For Reflection or Discussion

1. Polly and Peter's original decision to pursue sterilization was medically informed, theologically sound (at least in their circle of influence), and ethically defensible. How, then, could it have become morally unacceptable?

   ___ It didn't, it just felt that way.
   ___ Because it always was and they didn't know it until they were enlightened by this speaker.
   ___ Because group pressure greatly impacts moral values.
   ___ Actually, the real immorality here is the creation of guilt about their good faith decision.

2. Since Polly and Peter now see their original decision as sinful, what can they do to "get right with God"?

   ___ Polly should seek a reversal.
   ___ They might consider adoption, if they can't afford a reversal.
   ___ They should consider adoption, plus seek a reversal.
   ___ They should find a church more like their former one.
   ___ Nothing they can do will make them more right than simply accepting God's forgiveness on the basis of their faith.

3. Recall and share any instances you have encountered where there was either a subtle or overt sense of disap-

proval of a couple having or wanting a large family. While you're at it, try to define *large*.

4. Can you think of instances where Christians have imposed "onto the divine silence whatever interpretation best justifies what they are doing or might like to do"? What are the short-term and long-term results of this approach to Scripture, for individuals and the church at large?

5. Define *fruitfulness* in relation to God's design for marriage, and then more broadly in terms of his plan to expand the kingdom.

6. List reasons why a couple might decide that their "quiver" was full.

7. Think of situations other than medical reasons or possible danger where childlessness through sterilization might be justified on a biblical basis.

8. In the three years Judy and Sam had been married, they had produced three children. When a pastor visited after the birth of the third child, the conversation turned to large families. Judy's perspective was that the only way to proceed in this arena was to trust God that he would allow them to have the number of children he thought was right for them. How would you respond to her view?

9. Twice in Genesis these words occur: "Be fruitful and increase in number and fill the earth. . . ." To what degree is this command binding on Christians today?

___ Not at all, it was given to Adam and Noah, not to us.

___ Not at all, because it's in the Old Testament.

___ Somewhat, though it seems like the earth is pretty full.

___ It's binding on whoever wants it to bind them.
___ It's only a suggestion, not a command.
___ It's a principle that must be interpreted by other
texts.

10. Develop a set of principles related to sterilization from 1
Cor. 6: 19-20 and 7:4. Identify the main differences between
these principles and secular thinking.

11. Can you improve this statement: "As God's servants, and
as good stewards of our procreative capacities we will seek
to glorify him by raising up as godly offspring the quiver
full of children he has already given us. To better provide
for their physical, emotional, and spiritual needs, we
believe it is morally acceptable in his sight to seek permanent sterilization."

12. Review the policy you began to develop earlier, and see if
you can finalize it now.

Checklist for Decision Making

The following checklist might be helpful in reaching your personal decision about sterilization.

Gather information

___ I understand the procedures involved and what they accomplish.

___ I am aware of the costs and how they will be paid.

___ I understand that this procedure should be considered irreversible.

___ I understand the medical risks.

___ I understand the psychological risks.

___ If this is for a medical reason, I have sought a second opinion.

___ By this date _____ my decision should be made.

Ethical factors

My worldview as I make this decision is:

___ secular
___ Christian
___ mixed

The ethical principles guiding me are:

___ doing good
___ not doing harm
___ self-determination
___ God is sovereign
___ justice
___ stewardship

___ sanctity of life
___ suffering has purpose
___ eternity exists

As I understand the positions, secular ethics would allow me to:

_____

_____

_____

As I understand the positions, Christian ethics would allow me to:

_____

_____

_____

Theological principles
The Roman Catholic tradition helped me see that:

_____

_____

_____

The Protestant positions helped me see that:

_____

_____

_____

Biblical texts to consider:
___ Gen. 1:28; 9:1
___ Ps. 127:3-5; 128:1-4
___ Mal. 2:15
___ 1 Cor. 6:19, 20; 7:4
___ 1 Tim. 5:14

___ Gen. 2:24; Eph. 5:31-33
___ Matt. 19:13-15
___ John 15:1-8
___ Rom. 12:1-2
___ 1 Tim. 5:8
___ Heb. 4:12

Spiritual factors

As a result of searching Scripture to discern God's perspective on this, I have found:

_____

_____

_____

Having allowed Scripture to discern the thoughts and intentions of my heart, I believe these are my true motives for wanting to go ahead:

___ More children would be a physical hardship.
___ More children would be a financial burden.
___ More children would keep us from nurturing the children we have.
___ I am worried about genetic factors.
___ I want more time for myself.
___ If we have any more kids, my career will suffer.
___ I don't really like kids, now that I have some.
___ I'm too old to become a new parent.
___ Our quiver is full.
___ This will improve my relationship with my spouse.
___ It would be the only way to honor God and the children we already have.
___ Other:

_____

_____

_____

Relational factors

My spouse and I are in settled agreement that God would not under any circumstances want us to have another child.

I have sought the input of trusted advisors, including:

parents, who said:

other family members, who said:

pastor, who said:

other church leaders, who said:

non-church spiritual advisor(s), who said:

friends, who said:

If I proceed with this and am later tempted toward regret, I believe I will have involved enough trusted, spiritually minded people in this decision to affirm that I made this decision in good faith, with a clear conscience before God.

Affirmation

I believe that the position below is as medically informed, ethically defensible, theologically sound, and morally acceptable as I can develop at this time, and I affirm that I have reached it with the full agreement of my spouse.

This is what I believe regarding elective sterilization:

_____

_____

_____

_____

_____

_____

_____

Signed:_____

Date: _____

Signature of Spouse:_____

Notes

Chapter One: A Dilemma with Names and Faces

1. "As Birth-Control Options in the United States Dwindle, More Married Women Turn to Sterilization," *Scientific American* (July 1990) 18.
2. Ibid.
3. "UN Surveys Global Sex, Fertility Trends," *Boston Globe* (June 25, 1992) 85.

Chapter Two: Medically Informed

1. D. Wolfers and H. Wolfers. *Vasectomy and Vasectomania.* (Manchester, England: C. Nicholls, 1974).
2. A. J. Ochsner. "Surgical Treatment of Habitual Criminals," *Journal of the American Medical Association,* (1889) 32:867.
3. Ibid.

Chapter Three: Ethically Defensible

1. T. L. Beauchamp and J. F. Childress. *Principles of Biomedical Ethics,* 3rd ed. (New York: Oxford, 1989).
2. A. R. Jonsen. *The New Medicine & the Old Ethics.* (Cambridge, Mass.: Harvard, 1990).
3. "Ethical Considerations in Sterilization." (Washington, D.C.: American College of Obstetricians and Gynecologists, Sept. 1989) Committee Opinion Number 73.
4. R. H. Blank. *Fertility Control: New Techniques, New Policy Issues.* (New York: Greenwood, 1991) 48, 49.
5. Pope Paul VI. *Humanae Vitae: Encyclical Letter of His Holiness on the Regulation of Birth.* Cited by S. E. Lammers and A. Verhey in *On Moral Medicine.* (Grand Rapids: Eerdmans, 1987).

6. J. Grundel *Zur Problematik der operativen Sterilisation in Katholischen Krankenhausern.* Cited by R. A. McCormick in *Notes on Moral Theology, 1981-1989.* (New York: University of America) 84.

7. J. T. Noonan. "The History of Contraception: Seven Choices." Cited by S. F. Spiker, W. B. Bondeson, H. T. Engelhart, eds. in *The Contraceptive Ethos.* (Boston: Reidel, 1987).

8. D. H. Smith. *Health and Medicine in the Anglican Tradition.* (New York: Crossroad, 1986).

9. J. J. Davis. *Evangelical Ethics.* (Phillipsburg, N.J.: Presbyterian and Reformed, 1985) 44.

10. K. L. Vaux. *Health and Medicine in the Reformed Tradition.* (New York: Crossroad, 1984).

11. M. E. Marty. *Health and Medicine in the Lutheran Tradition.* (New York: Crossroad, 1986).

12. E. B. Holifield. *Health and Medicine in the Methodist Tradition.* (New York: Crossroad, 1986).

13. N. E. Himes. *Medical History of Contraception.* (New York: Gamut, 1963) xiv.

14. R. H. Harrison, ed. *Encyclopedia of Biblical & Christian Ethics.* (Nashville: Thomas Nelson, 1992).

15. "Is Birth Control Christian?" *Christianity Today* (Nov. 11, 1991)34.

16. R. C. Van Leeuwen.*Christianity Today* (Nov. 11, 1991) 37.

17. C. F. H. Henry. *Birth Control and the Christian.* (Wheaton, Ill.: Tyndale, 1969) Foreword.

Chapter Four: Theologically Sound

1. For Jewish perspectives see "Birth Control," *Encyclopedia Judaica.* (New York: Macmillan, 1971) 4:1054. See also D. M. Feldman. *Marital Relations, Birth Control, and Abortion in Jewish Law.* (New York: Schocken, 1968) 243ff. For Eastern Orthodox perspectives, see Chrysostom Zaphiris. "The Morality of Contraception: An Eastern Orthodox Opinion," *Journal of Ecumenical Studies II,* 1974) 661-90.

2. Norman P. Tanner, ed. *Decrees of the Ecumenical Councils.* (New York: Sheed and Ward, 1990) 1:6.

3. "Sterilization," *New Catholic Encyclopedia.* (New York: McGraw Hill, 1967) 13:704; See also John T. Noonan, Jr. *Contraception: A History of Its Treatment by the Catholic Theologians and Canonists.* (Cambridge: Harvard, 1966).

4. Thomas J. O'Donnell. *Morals in Medicine.* (Westminster, Md.: Newman, 1959) 79.

5. Ibid, 132.

6. Ibid.

7. Charles J. McFadden. *Medical Ethics,* 6th ed. (Philadelphia: F. A. Davis, 1967) 307.

8. Benedict M. Ashley and Kevin D. O'Rourke. *Healthcare Ethics: A Theological Analysis.* 6th ed. St. Louis: Catholic Health Assn. 1989) 272

9. Richard A. McCormick. "Sterilization and Theological Method," *Theological Studies* (1976) 37:473-475. See also Bernard Haring. *Medical Ethics.* (South Bend, Ind.: Notre Dame: 1973) 62.

10. Robert M. Cooper. "Vasectomy and the Good of the Whole," *Anglican Theological Review* (1972) 54:97.

11. Ibid, 98.

12. Dietrich Bonhoeffer. *Ethics.* Eberhard Bethge, ed. (New York: Macmillan, 1955) 181.

13. Ibid.

14. Joseph Fletcher. *Morals and Medicine.* (Princeton, N.J.: Princeton University, 1954) 145.

15. Ibid.

16. Ibid.

17. Walter O. Spitzer and Carlyle L. Saylor, eds. *Birth Control and the Christian.* (Wheaton: Tyndale, 1969) 257-98. The affirmation statement is on pages 27, 28. In 1985 The Christian Medical and Dental Society passed a far more conservative official statement opposing abortion.

18. J. N. D. Anderson. *Issues of Life and Death.* (Downers Grove, Ill.: InterVarsity, 1976) 71.

19. Ibid.

20. Ibid, 75.

21. Franklin E. Payne, Jr. *Making Biblical Decisions.* (Escondido, Calif.: Hosanna House, 1959) 52. For a position similar to that of Payne's, see John Jefferson David, *Evangelical Ethics,* 2d ed. (Phillipsburg, N.J.: Presbyterian and Reformed, 1993) 41, 42.

22. Payne, 54.

23. Ibid.

24. Ibid, 182.

25. Ibid, 183.

26. Ibid.

27. Peter C. Craigie. *The Book of Deuteronomy.* (Grand Rapids: Eerdmans, 1976) 297.

28. H. W. F. Saggs in Craigie: 297 n6.

29. Robert H. Gundry. *Matthew: A Commentary on His Literary and Theological Art.* (Grand Rapids: Eerdmans, 1982) 382.

30. Ibid, 383. See also W. C. Allen. *A Critical and Exegetical Commentary on the Gospel According to Saint Matthew,* 3rd ed. (Edinburgh: T & T Clark, 1912) 206.

31. Nahum Sarna. *The JPS Torah Commentary: Genesis.* (Philadelphia: Jewish Publication Society, 1989) 353 n23.

32. Gordon J. Wenham. *Word Biblical Commentary: Genesis 1-15*. (Waco, Tex.: Word, 1987) 33.

33. Ibid.

34. Ibid. The rabbis discussed the matter of family size. In relation to Genesis 1:28 it was said, "A man must not abstain from 'fruitfulness and increase' unless he already has children. The school of Shammai say, Two sons, but the school of Hillel say, A son and a daughter, because it says, 'Male and female He created them.' Mishnah *Yebamoth 6:6*.

In Plato's legislation for the ideal state, a minimum, of one boy and one girl were specified for each couple: *Laws* 11.930 cd, cited in Robert Garland, *The Greek Way of Life*. (Ithaca, N.Y.: Cornell University Press, 1990) 102.